Health And Fitness
Tips
That Will Change
Your Life

Create a healthy lifestyle from beginner
to winner with mind-set, diet, and
exercise habits

JimsHealthAndMuscle.com

Health And Fitness Tips
That Will Change Your Life

Create a healthy lifestyle from beginner to winner with mind-set, diet and exercise habits

JAMES ATKINSON

JIMSHEALTHANDMUSCLE.COM
PAPERBACK EDITION

PUBLISHED BY:
JBA publishing
http://www.jimshealthandmuscle.com
jim@jimshealthandmuscle.com

Book Proofing, Design & Layout by Papertrue

Fitness & Exercise Motivation
Copyright © 2017 by James Atkinson
All Rights Reserved.

ISBN- 978-0-9932791-6-4

DISCLAIMER

First published in 2017 / First printed in 2017
Printed in United Kingdom

TABLE OF CONTENTS

PREFACE

I can't begin to tell you how many times I have stood in this spot, feeling my biceps burn after a satisfying set of cable curls. I could feel my arms bulging and the hem of my t shirt straining around them. This is why I'm here; this is what I have built; and this is what I do.

Every January is the same – new faces in the gym, and by April, it will be back to just the usual crowd.

As I listen to the metal music pumping into my ears through the headphones that separate me from the distraction of conversation and social interaction, I scan the gym.

I make sure that the peak of my baseball cap serves as a partial shield for my gaze and a deterrent against useless conversation. I am serious about my training and don't need to be interrupted by fair-weather trainers.

There are more newcomers than ever this year, and I can tell that many have never been involved in fitness all their lives, and so, they don't know how hard this game is. Among the new faces, I notice a guy, probably in his mid-thirties; he's a big man who is out of shape and wears big, baggy clothes to match. I think of all of the work that I have put in and wonder – what is the difference between me and him?

Back to my training, I blast out another set of biceps cable curls. Pumped up again, my biceps are bulging and tight. I better stretch out the muscles; I smile to myself as I imagine my biceps tearing out of my skin from training too hard.

As I stretch out my arms to relax my biceps, I am drawn to my thirty-something new gym associate again. He's not wasting any time and appears to know what he's doing. He has a good routine going for himself and is working hard on a circuit using a mix of bodyweight and barbell exercises. He's working out in a quiet corner of the gym and has everything organised.

Taking note of this, I can immediately tell that this guy has a goal, a plan, work ethics; he wants his fitness results and is willing to work for them, and I respect this on a level that I am yet to understand.

Seeing this new trainer in a new light, I realise that he may well be the exception to the stereotype of "January gym start-ups".

This guy is different; it certainly appears that he has put in some work already with his planning, and his actions tell of his motivation and will to succeed. He most definitely stands out from the crowd.

I finish up my stretching and refocus on my own goals. I reach for my waiting bar and ready myself for another intense set.

Four weeks later, it's February. The days are still short, the heat of the sun still elusive, and the metal of the bar that I grip is ice cold, although that doesn't keep me from my gym sessions or my fitness goals.

As predicted, there are a fewer faces in the gym than the previous month. However, over the last few weeks, without fail, I have shared floor space and gym time with that new starter who had grabbed my attention earlier. He wears the same gym clothes and is still training in his unique circuit style with bodyweight and barbell exercises in a quiet corner of the gym. The weights on his bar have increased, he is doing more reps on his bodyweight exercises, and he looks more confident in his exercise delivery.

I pick up my bar and complete my set. I am also wearing the same clothes and doing the very exercise that I was doing the first time we were in the gym together.

As I stretch out my arms, I witness him finish one of his circuit sets. He stands tall with his hands on his hips, looks up to the ceiling as if he is challenging an unknown force, breathes deeply but calmly, and I can tell that he is already thinking about his next set.

He rolls his shoulders and makes eye contact with me. I give him a nod of acknowledgement, he returns the gesture, and we both fall back into our routines.

The month of May certainly lifts the mood of most people. I love this time of year: new life, the sun's warmth, and the promise of potential. Outside, everything is green, fresh, and new.

I walk into the gym to begin my session, and as soon as I step into the free weights area, I notice a familiar sight – It's the same guy that's been training since January. He is between sets and is stretching out his biceps. His gaze is fixed on a new comer of the gym, and he is obviously lost in thought. As he holds the stretch, he shakes the thoughts away, rolls his shoulders, and prepares for his next set.

The bar and dumbbells that he has around him are a lot heavier than they were a month or two ago. He is still wearing the same gym cloths that he had been wearing since he started; they are more faded, but they look like they are hanging off of him. It reminds me of my school days when my friend's mom would buy his school uniform two sizes too big for him as part of a money saving plan. This makes me smile, and at that moment, he catches my eye. I throw my arm high and give him a thumbs up from the other side of the gym; he smiles back at me and does the same. He looks at his push-up mat on the floor and assumes the starting position before getting started on his next set.

Several months earlier, I had asked myself, "What is the difference between this guy and me?" I now know the answer. The only difference is that he started training only a few years later than I did, and now, I can't ever imagine him being without it. He has earned some great results and overcame many challenges. I know that it's not just the few hours that I see him in the gym every week that has made all the difference; from my personal experience, I know that he has had to make major lifestyle changes to be where he is right now. I respect him immensely for this – more than he will ever come to know.

This was my personal experience; it happened about ten years ago, and it changed my outlook on beginners to fitness. I will admit that I was a bit arrogant back then, and I took the lessons that I had learnt on my own fitness journey for granted. I was absorbed in bodybuilding and prioritised and focused on my own goals rather than helping others. I had never actually spoken to this guy; but he is one of the few people that had made an impression on me in that gym. I now train at a different establishment and often wonder how he is getting along. I also regret not going over and congratulating him on his fitness achievements since he had accomplished what so many people try but fail to do.

The point of this story is to demonstrate that I completely empathise with the struggle that comes with weight-loss and fitness results. I believe that everyone deserves the opportunity to achieve their goals, however unobtainable they may seem; and I'm here to turn this mountain into a gentle gradient that you hardly even notice.

As our friend exhibited, it wasn't just his efforts in the gym that earned him his results; I know that this was just the tip of the iceberg. My aim for this book is to give you a blueprint that will allow you to achieve results similar to our friend by giving you easy to follow tweaks and fitness tips that you can apply to your lifestyle and can implement every two weeks.

In my opinion, weight-loss and fitness results are only worth working for if they are long-term and sustainable. As my father and grandfather always told me –

"Nothing that's worth having is EVER easy to get."

This is never more true when it comes to earning weight-loss and fitness results. In this book, however, I will help you make it as easy as possible by drawing on my own experience of over twenty years of trial and error, failure to success. You will be way ahead of the game and have your best chance of ensuring your journey to fitness and weight-loss triumph is as painless and smooth as possible.

Let's get started!

INTRODUCTION

In the summer of 2016 I published a book called *Fitness & Exercise Motivation*. The book had done very well on its launch, and it has been connecting me with some great people around the world ever since. Every time I hit the publish button on a book, I am unsure of how my work will be received, but the reaction to *Fitness & Exercise Motivation* has been very reassuring to me. This book and its audio version has actually helped its readers and listeners change their lives. It's so good to be a small part of their fitness success.

I always like offering extra help and pointers to everyone and welcome messages to my inbox or through social media; I have already assisted plenty of readers/listeners tweak exercise plans or aspects of a generic plan to better suit their personal goals.

In the wake of *Fitness & Exercise Motivation*, many readers/listeners have developed a high level of motivation to attain their goals, created a plan, and started following it; nevertheless, some common questions reached me asking about more specific steps to further their development.

One day in December 2016, I spent a solid four hours answering emails from readers. Although this may seem like a tedious task to most, it's an extremely rewarding part of this game to me. That day, the idea for *Health & Fitness Tips That will Change your Life* was conceived. If you are highly motivated to start on a fitness journey, you would want to harness that motivation to see that your goals are realised; it may include programmes for fat loss, stamina development, strength building or something more activity oriented, such as running a marathon, cycle races, or triathlons. The less hurdles that you have to jump on your road to success, the easier it will be for you.

I believe that anyone can attain a fitness goal if they have the right ingredients in the right measures. To be clear, this statement is not coming from someone who is genetically gifted for athletics, is naturally confident, is an academic success, or a guy that had had an excessive amount of help. It comes from a guy who misses more than he hits; a guy who has never been confident in his abilities, despite his achievements as a guy who was in the "special" class for English at school; so, in other words, the statement is coming from a guy who is below average or average at best in general terms.

Over the last twenty years and more, I have been skinny and weak, a long-distance runner, fat and unfit, and then a competing bodybuilder. I am a qualified fitness coach and personal trainer and have been through the mill when it comes to personal fitness. I now have a balanced healthy lifestyle, which is the direct result of my journey. But, why should it take you more than twenty years to hit your fitness goals and learn how to live a healthy lifestyle?

This is where I can help you. In this book, I will outline the fundamental building blocks that are essential for fitness success, and I will show you exactly how to implement them. I will demonstrate the exact steps that I would take in order to compete in a triathlon, run a marathon, or compete in a bodybuilding competition if I had been sitting around watching television, playing computer games, and eating pizza for the last twenty years – and all of this will only take around twenty-five steps.

Every success story in fitness has a beginning, and it is very rarely a straight smooth road to the finish line; it's okay to fall over or hit a roadblock on your way, but as long as you cross that finish line, you will be a winner. My aim it to help you attain your specific fitness goal or at least be very close to attaining them in around a year. Whatever happens, if you follow this plan, you won't look back.

GRAB YOUR BONUS

Although this book's focus is not entirely on the physical exercise part of the fitness and lifestyle puzzle, physical exercise is in fact one of the major players.

To thank you for your purchase, I would like to offer you a fully illustrated and entirely free PDF download created by myself to give you a head start and use in conjunction with this book. This will give you the tools to start a quick, but highly effective, workout routine from your own home.

Simply click the link below or copy the following URL into your web browser. I will be there to greet you via a video message and explain more about this quick start-up routine.

jimshealthandmuscle.com/free-training/

The exercises that I have chosen in this routine are perfect for beginners and can be used right up to expert training. They are very versatile, and you will soon learn how to use them in many different ways for different fitness results.

I'm really looking forward to our training; so, I'll see you on the inside!

ONE

HEALTH CHECK

Before you embark on any fitness routine, please consult your doctor.

1. Do not exercise if you are unwell.
2. Stop if you feel pain, and if the pain does not subside, please visit your doctor.
3. Do not exercise if you have taken alcohol or had a large meal in the last few hours.
4. If you are taking medication, please check with your doctor to make sure it is okay for you to exercise.
5. If in doubt at all, please check with your doctor first. It may be helpful to ask for a blood pressure, cholesterol, and weight check. You can then have these tested again in a few months after starting your exercise routine to see the benefits.

TWO

WHERE ARE THE FITNESS TIPS?

Although the main draw for this book may be the list of tips that you can start implementing right away to begin to develop your fitness, work on your amazing fat loss journey, and start living a healthy happy life in a body that you are proud of, there are some building blocks that need to be laid first to help with your mind-set shift.

It's all well and good skipping the first section of this book and heading right to the actionable steps, but by doing so, you may miss out on vital information.

I, for one, am a guy who likes to know why I am doing what I am doing, or why something happens the way it does. If I am told that a thirty minute jog is far better for fat burning than a short sprint session, I want to know why. Why does a slow comfortable jog burn more fat than two twenty second sprint sessions that are likely to leave me feeling completely exhausted? This type of knowledge is second nature to me now but there was a time when it wasn't. I've grown to realise that the more you know about why things happen in relation to your goals, the better you are able to work with the tools that you have; you will become more efficient and better equipped to reach these achievements.

Therefore, before we jump right into the twenty-five fitness tips, I would like to share some theories and advice that has been gleaned from my own experiences. During my twenty years' involvement, I have achieved some lofty goals in the health and fitness world, and it has been far from being an easy ride. If I were to start from scratch knowing what I know now, it would take me a fraction of the time to get to where I wanted to be.

Over the years, I have come to realise that it's not just the physical training that you do, the food that you eat, or even the mental conditioning that you endure that carry you to success; it's the right

9

balance of all the three and knowing how to work with these pieces of the puzzle and turning them to your advantage.

In this book, I will show you the how and why of every suggested fitness tip so that you are not left guessing. Although there are twenty-five specific fitness tips that you can follow outlined in this book, which will span over a year, I will also guide you in modifying these to make your own plan more suited to your individual needs.

Whichever way you decide to play it, You will have the next one year of fitness routine planned out by the time you finish this book, and you will be on the road to achieving the level of fitness and healthy living that you have always wanted. If you do finish this book and still happen to have questions, please remember that I am always happy to help you out further; so, don't be a stranger and just give me a shout.

So how does this guide work?

This guide is designed to help you systematically and gradually change the three biggest aspects of your life that have the most influence over your fitness, health, and wellbeing: mind-set, diet and exercise. If you are unfit, overweight, have low self-esteem, confused about where to start, or just feel that you want to make positive changes to your body and mind, this guide offers the blueprint that you need to start with.

Each small change will fit into one of the three categories listed above. Instead of taking all of these fitness tips and putting them to test on your first day, you should plan out the next full year in advance and implement a single change on a biweekly basis. This way, you only have to focus on a single task at a time. I wouldn't suggest making a change every week, since a single week can fly past you, and the change that you were working on might not have taken hold before you are faced with another challenge. There are more chances that you will be overwhelmed if you go for weekly changes. However, this obviously depends on individual circumstances.

I will reiterate the importance of longevity at this point. Some of these fitness tips may feel like they are hardly worth following, but the concept is solid. As long as you stick to the plan and keep up with your changes, you will get your health and fitness results.

If you follow this, you will foster positive habits and strengthen your mental attitude.

The guide is split into two sections:

Section 1 – In this section, we will look at the theory behind some of the practicals by highlighting the importance of the most commonly overlooked aspects of heath, weight-loss, and fitness development by drawing on some examples of real-life situations and experiences that have been the deciding factors in my own success.

Section 2 – This section not only lists the practical fitness tips that you can follow directly for your next year of weight-loss and fitness, but it also explains why you would make them in the order that is advised. Each change will be related to either mental development, diet, or exercise and will have suggestions on how you can build on this change or devise your own.

THREE

MENTAL HEALTH AND FITNESS

A healthy mind starts with a healthy body; a healthy body promotes a healthy mind.

An important part of achieving fitness goals is to have a good state of mental health. However, partaking in exercise sessions and having health aspiration doesn't just require good mental health. The whole process develops mental health in a positive way, and I feel that fitness and health plans are widely underrated and overlooked when it comes to their effectiveness in remedying mental health issues.

This is a subject that I have never written about before. Although mind-set has always been a major part of my works, I have never directly addressed the influence that fitness training and its resultant effect can have over conditions such as depression. I had always felt that I was unqualified to delve into this area and that the thoughts and opinions I have on the subject should be kept to my own counsel or left to qualified psychiatrists.

Reflecting on this, the books I write and the training programs that I design are intended to help people who are struggling in one way or another with health and fitness or are looking for new ways to train for better results. Since this information is based on my personal experiences, sharing the pitfalls and mistakes that I have made on my journey will help the readers avoid these errors themselves and essentially get to the finish line a lot quicker than I ever did.

As an observer of my own life and the positive impact that health and fitness has, and has had, on it, I can unequivocally state that regular exercise and a healthy diet can beat or drastically alleviate feelings of depression, low self-esteem, and other mental ailments or conditions.

How do I know this for certain? Well, as with all of the other training writings of personal involvement, I have experienced times of self-doubt, low self-esteem, and general feelings of depression. It may come as a surprise to many that I would confess to such a thing, but in my opinion, everyone has feelings of depression at some point in their lives; some people are prey to depression and have a hard time coming out of it allowing it to control their entire existence, while the other set realise that they are depressed and proactively try to come out of its grip.

As far back as I can remember, I have completed at least three exercise sessions per week. Obviously, there have been a few exceptions, but in general terms, this is my benchmark for minimum training sessions per week. If I don't hit these exercise sessions and go too long without training, some strange things happen to my mind-set.

- When I look in the mirror, I start to perceive myself differently. I begin to see myself with less muscle or more body fat than I actually have.
- I feel that I am letting myself down.
- My self-esteem dwindles.
- I have feelings of "What's the point of training or doing anything?" creep in or feelings of hopelessness in general.
- I lose my ambition.
- I feel that a single training session has absolutely no power to change any of this... but, I *know* that it will.

As soon as I am at the gym, all of this negativity goes away, and I am recharged with positivity.

If this works for me, I am sure that it will work for others who have serious mental health conditions.

As I mentioned earlier, I'm not a professional psychoanalyst, and I have no qualifications on the subject, but I do feel empathy towards others who struggle with mental health conditions, especially if the condition is destructive and holds them back from their potential.

It shouldn't be that way, and I believe that everyone who suffers from depression or other physiological problems such as addiction should start with a health and fitness plan.

An obsessive or addictive nature is linked to depression. I have an addictive nature too, and I believe everyone does to a certain extent. However, I overcome bad or damaging addictions by replacing them with "healthy" or "constructive" addictions.
It is obviously not healthy to be obsessed or addicted to anything; but the point that I am making is that it is possible to channel any addiction or obsession that is negative into one that is positive, and this is a fundamental foundation block for building a strong healthy mind, which in turn will be the foundation for building a strong healthy body.

It is hard work to be positive all the time! Although, if you do it for long enough, like the building of any habit, it will become easy or even your second nature.
There are many personal experiences that I could share to help hammer this point home, but a fairly recent one springs to my mind.

I have been cycling to the gym for several years now. It is a six-mile round trip; I cycle around three miles there, train with weights, and then cycle back.

A major portion of this route runs along a busy main road that also has several busy junctions and roundabouts. Unfortunately, there is a small section of this road that does not have an adjacent cycle path; only a pedestrian access. One particular morning, I went through the usual ritual of filling my water bottle, throwing on my gym kit, putting my backpack on, wheeling my bike out, and setting off for my gym session. It was a nice enough day for a bike ride, and the roads were fairly quiet. In less than a minute, I had reached the junction at which I would turn onto the main road that I needed to follow in order to reach the gym. Please remember that I am from the UK, so we drive on the left. This is the stretch that is missing a cycle path. I peddled along this road just like I had done countless times before. About half a mile on, I neared a junction that fed traffic onto the road from my left, and as I approached, I noticed a nice-looking car heading ahead to join the road in front of me. As I got even closer, I trusted that this car would stop as it was my right of way.

"He must have seen me," I remember thinking, "there's no way he hasn't seen me."

As I crossed the junction, *Bang!* The car seemed to speed up and slammed right into my side. I bounced off the bonnet and was knocked into the filter lane that was designed for traffic turning right. Luckily, there was nothing coming.

I think it's fair to say that this is a pretty negative experience; so, with the assumption that this is true, on analysing my own thought process throughout the incident, it's quite amazing to look back at how I reacted.

A lot seemed to happen instinctively in a split second; somehow, I was aware of what was going on. I accepted that I had just been hit by a car; yes, some curse words did come out of my mouth. I had made a mental note that I needed to get up as soon as I could after I landed because I didn't want to get hit by oncoming traffic. I also made a note to land as cleanly as possible to limit the damage. Thus, as soon as I hit the deck, I worked on getting up on my feet. A quick check, and I found that my leg was a bit stiff; but it worked. I had a hole in the palm of my glove from the initial contact with the tarmac, but that seemed to be all. I scanned the road as I got up on my feet and scooped up all of the parts of my bike that were scattered (This only turned out to be my front light; but for a small thing, it had broken into a surprising number of pieces). I picked up my bike and wheeled it to the side of the road.

A couple of pedestrians on their morning dog walk stood open-mouthed at the other side of the road and after a short time shouted across to see if I was okay. I shouted back, "It's all good" as I gave them a thumbs up.

They stood for a while longer, probably wondering if they should do something. The guy who was driving the car had pulled over, and he was apparently very shaken. He was still sitting in the driver's seat with his hands fixed on the steering wheel. At this point, I had felt that I needed to be the one to reassure him and make sure he was okay.

I walked over to the passenger side and opened the door. In hindsight, this may have put him under more stress as I didn't look like the most savoury of characters, wearing a black beanie hat, fingerless gloves, a full beard, and a heavy thermal overcoat. I would have, however, fitted in nicely standing around a burning trash can, sipping from a bottle wrapped in a brown paper bag under a bridge in a dubious part of town.

"Don't worry," I said, making sure that I had a smile on my face to put him at ease and assure him that I wasn't going to drag him out of the car, "Everything's okay. Not too sure about your car though."

"Are you okay?" he asked.

"Yeah, it could have been worse," I replied.

He got out of the vehicle, and we both walked to its front.

There were two dents in the bonnet – A big "soft" dent where I had landed, which could probably have been easily fixed by just pushing the underside of it. There was another dent where the handle bar of my bike had hit. This was a real dent and had taken off some of the paint.

"Ooooh, that's gonna be tricky to sort out," I said with a concerned grimace.

The driver was now more at ease – which was nice to see – and I could tell that he could understand the measure of my outlook on this situation.

"I've only just had it washed too," he said.

One thing that I was aware of was that he never apologised. There was no doubt that it was his fault, and this made me realise that he may not have been as shaken up by the incident as I had first thought. Its common knowledge that apologising is admitting fault, and he was obviously thinking clearly enough to know this and act accordingly.

Realising this, I decided to maintain my upbeat attitude and be on my way as soon as I could. Although, I wasn't willing to offer any more sympathy to the car.

"Looks like it's a trip to the body work shop next then, I guess? I think the bikes okay... just the light is smashed. Like I said, it could have been a lot worse. Anyway, I better get on"

I headed over to my bike, adjusted my backpack again, picked the bike up, and continued my ride to the gym. I was training legs that day, and that's an important session not to miss.

It turned out that the bike was damaged – the back wheel was buckled, and the gears were ruined. It was the bike mentioned in the preface of my book *Fitness & Exercise Motivation*; so, if you have read that one, you will know that it was a hand-me-down from a good friend, and the sentimental value far outweighed the monetary value.

I have told this story to several people, and every one of them told me that they would have handled the situation differently, and I'm sure that many folks that read about it here would have too.
When I look back at this and try and figure out why I instinctively acted the way that I did, I think it all boils down to my general attitude and the way that I have developed my mental health over many years of tough physical exertions.

Challenges and adversity are a major part of life; so, if you can accept this and confront any negative encounter with a positive attitude, you will have cracked it.
Yes, I know it's very easy to say, "Just be positive" as we all know that actions are the harder part, but I know from my own experience that developing strength in the form of mental health is no different from developing strength in any other muscle of the body. You just have to know what exercises to do, and this does not happen overnight. For example, if you decide that you wanted to build your quad muscles up by doing squats, but you've never even done bodyweight squats before and right away stepped into a squat rack, took a loaded bar on your shoulders, and began your first twelve reps of 100kg, you would probably have damaged your knees, your back, and be lying on the floor underneath the weights and the bar before you even completed your first rep.
In reality, to do this you would have to –

- learn the squatting movement using only your bodyweight and maybe even some form of support
- perfect the movement
- increase the number of reps
- introduce the bar
- increase the weight and reps until you hit your goal
- work on your nutrition to aid correct recovery from training sessions and ensure progression
- be consistent with your progression and training session

This would take a good four to six months in the most optimistic of estimates.

Therefore, if developing mental health is the same as building physical health; in my opinion, the same amount of work is needed for progressive, positive development in this area, as much as it is needed for the physical. In many cases, mental strength training is far more important. That's why, in this book, there will be a big focus on the training of the mind along with everything else.

It's almost impossible to achieve outstanding fitness and weight-loss results without a strong, healthy mind. Again, the very nature of the fitness journey itself, and the challenges that must be conquered, offers everything that is needed in the strengthening of the mind. Thus, developing one of these traits will inadvertently cause a positive by-product of development for the other; but, if you are aware of this and work on increasing both at the same time, you will be in very good standing indeed, and you will almost definitely see the benefits that this training offers in all aspects of your life.

FOUR

YES! TOO MANY POTATOES CAN RUIN YOUR DAY

It's no secret that a lot of a little makes a lot. Moreover, the premise of "habit stacking" or creating lots of small positive habits that will make huge differences in the long term is widespread. If you are unfamiliar with this concept, here is one of my favourite analogies that I created to explain weight-loss to my clients.

Let's imagine that you want to lose forty-five pounds of body fat (this is just over three stone for anyone who deals in stone rather than pounds), but this weight is represented by a big bag of potatoes that is constantly strapped around you. Right away, you can see how much of an inconvenience this would be. You would have to carry these potatoes around with you wherever you go, find a way to sleep around them, go to work with them; even if you had to go out with your friends, the potatoes would go along with you – they are basically a part of you. To say that this is hard work would be a bit of an understatement. We won't even go into what you might look like when you are out about town or grocery shopping; after all, this is a lot of potatoes.

The only way that you would be able to get rid of this cumbersome weight that is making your life so hard would be to shed them one at a time. But, there is a catch! You can only take one potato out of the bag every week, and that is only if you have completed all of your planned workout sessions and have adhered to your healthy eating plan. Your reward for putting in the required effort is taking one potato out of the bag every week. Of course, some potatoes are bigger than others, so you may be even luckier on some weeks.

On the other hand, if you don't stick to your diet and exercise plans, an extra potato is added to your bag! The last thing you need is for this bag of spuds to become an even bigger burden.

The most challenging weeks by far are going to be the early ones. In this time, not only do you have this outrageously large bag of potatoes to haul around with you, you also have to stick to a new diet; this comes with a new food prep experience, which in turn takes up more of your time before you master it. You have to get yourself (and the potatoes) to the gym for your training sessions; and of course, these sessions will be a bit harder due to the extra weight; on top of all this, you still have to hold down a job and carry out all duties that come along with owning a house and having a family.

And, what do you get for a full week of this torture? The "satisfaction" of removing one single potato from the huge bag that has become the bane of your life.

Granted, this will be an extremely challenging task, not only from a physical point of view, but even more so from the mental aspect. However, if you were actually doing this and a single potato was removed every week, there will eventually come a point when you can actually feel the bag becoming lighter and more manageable. There will even be a point when you can see an end to it; when you can count the few weeks left; and finally, there will come a time when you reach the very last potato and relinquish your burden entirely.

The beauty of this analogy is that although it sounds silly and far-fetched, it's so very similar to a real weight-loss undertaking. All of the ingredients are the same – in real life, you should only expect to lose a small amount of weight per week, and the payoff may seem unfair at the beginning. It will be hard to start with; there are many changes to make; and it can become overwhelming. A feeling of hopelessness is not uncommon. The physical challenges will be tough, and the mental ones fierce. Though, once you progress through the weeks, things will start to change. The once big challenges will become "normal tasks" for you, and you will begin to take them in your stride. You will form solid, positive routines that will become a part of your everyday life; your mental strength will improve along with your physical health. You will be carrying less weight in the form of body fat, and your results will serve to motivate you even further. Ultimately, you will have hit your goals, achieved success, and developed great fortitude of character.

I find it immensely satisfying when I am able to convince someone who previously had the "I want to lose 45pounds, and I want to lose it yesterday" approach that it takes time and effort to hit their weight-loss goals. Understanding and accepting that there will be some very tough challenges ahead is the true starting point for fitness success and especially for weight-loss accomplishments.

Unfortunately, the whole struggle of the "carrying potatoes" analogy is not the typical approach for the newly motivated beginner to fitness and weight-loss. If the beginner can appreciate that results take time, hard work, and consistency to achieve and that it is a gradual process rather than all-out potato-sack-emptying, another common pitfall can then be avoided too.

Okay, so achieving fitness and weight-loss results can be hard work, and it takes time; but, there is no need to make it harder by taking the "all changes at once" attitude. This approach might work for someone who is very strong-willed and focused, but it is a lot harder than the slow burn. I wouldn't really advise it for most as this is what tends to happen – Sunday night comes and tomorrow is the big day. This is when the beginner will start. First thing on Monday morning, he will get up an hour early and go for his first run. After the run, he will have a healthy breakfast made in a juicer. At work, there will be a healthy lunch; all of the usual cups of coffee will be replaced with plenty of water. On the way home from work, he will visit the gym for a quick resistance training session, and to round off a great day, there will be a healthy meal of steamed broccoli, brown rice, and boiled chicken breast.

So, our fitness beginner, for as far back as he can remember and up until now, has lived a very sedentary life with no concern for healthy eating and the preparation that can come with it. For him, exercise, physical and mental challenges, not to mention the "caffeine crutch" that he has grown to depend on, is going to have a hard time when the impact of all these big changes that he has initiated start to stack up and work to beat him and his motivation down. Once you lose your motivation, it gets a lot harder. Thus, it's risky to gamble with this motivation; you wouldn't want to lose it now that you have it. The motivation that has developed in someone is the driving force of every single fitness endeavour; it is this force that actually turns thoughts and plans into actions that ultimately gets the ball rolling. This motivation is an exceptionally powerful thing when it comes to earning fitness results, but it is extremely fragile. This valuable resource will be sapped away in a very short time if you don't use it wisely.

This approach is normal, and it is hardly surprising when you consider the modern "next-day delivery" culture that we live in. So, what if it was possible to preserve this prized motivation and make the process a lot more comfortable, while also dropping the vertical gradient of the challenge curve to a barely noticeable incline?

It is, in fact, possible. But, one of the keys to making this happen is convincing the beginner that it will take time, many small, consistent changes, and that the toughest part will be the beginning.

FIVE

THE TOP 5 BIG MISTAKES

The main aim of this book is to guarantee that you have the best chance of fitness success. To ensure this success, I would like to reveal some of the most common big mistakes that are made when starting out. If you make any of these mistakes at the outset, you will be putting more challenges in the way of your final goal. This task is hard enough anyway, so you would want to eliminate as many hurdles and barriers as possible.

Here are my top five big mistakes that you should be aware of before starting out:

#1 - Thinking that it will be easy or quick

We live in an age of instant gratification – you can watch new movies on your 80 inch smart TV by pressing a few buttons; you can cook a frozen lasagne in a few minutes; you can get next-day or even same-day delivery on all types of products. I could order that 80 inch smart TV right now from my laptop and have it delivered to my house in a few hours. I can even shop for groceries from my laptop and have them delivered to my door!

When you think about it, there isn't really a whole lot that you can't get right away these days. So, when it comes to fitness and weight-loss results, a modern guy or girl that has no prior knowledge of what it really takes will want to reap what they have sown before they have even sown it.

The best way to avoid this misconception is to make sure that you understand that it's not an overnight process and that it will take more than just a few weeks of staying true to your plans to get great results. You should have faith that the longer you stay consistent, the easier it will get, and the more efficient your body will become and then, it will take less effort to get the same result. However, to get to this stage, you have to earn it.

Back when I was taking on new clients for personal training, I was approached by a girl who was in her late teens. She was entirely new to fitness, very overweight, and uninitiated in the way of exercise and nutrition. From the first twenty seconds of our initial meeting, it was very clear that there was a lot of work to be done, and I felt that with her current mind-set, this was an impossible task. It takes a *lot* for me to say that something is impossible; even today, I am hard-pushed to say that someone "can't" do something. To be honest, I admit to being over-optimistic in my overall outlook. However, in this instance, I had little hope.

We sat down, and I asked her a few questions about her goals and aspirations. The simple fact was that she wanted to slim down and have a healthier body in general. After a few more questions about her general lifestyle, I had a good idea of where to start with the exercise and told her, "I think the best thing that we can do right now is to do a three training session per week plan to start with. We will do a mix of light cardio, treadmill, cross trainer or bike – that kind of thing. And I also want to add some basic resistance training... with some of the dumb-bells and..."

"Can I just stop you there?" she interrupted, "I don't want to get a six-pack or anything like that."

This actually put me on the back foot, and this statement brought about the true import of this young ladies naivety. This was actually a defining moment for me as a personal trainer. Up until this point, I knew that a certain mind-set was required to attain even the most subtle of fitness progressions, and I assumed that everyone else did too. However, I was not prepared for this kind of a challenge as a personal trainer. Because of her lack of understanding of what it really takes to make physical changes, I know that she would not have been as reassured as she should have been by my answer: "Erm... It actually takes a lot more work than you would think to get any type of muscle definition, and abs are one of the trickiest parts of the body to develop visually. People who have six packs don't have them by accident."

I did want to go into an explanation of the benefits of weight training for fat loss and the theories behind it, but to be honest, these few words had taken away a lot of my hope and motivation. It wasn't exactly the words that frustrated me so much, but it was what they represented.

I had been into extreme fitness for over ten years at this point, and I had always *known* that everybody knew that weight-loss, muscle-building, or any kind of impressive fitness result takes hard work and dedication. I also *knew* that everybody appreciated the efforts that I had put into my own training to have what I had; and this is why they sought me out for personal training sessions. It turned out that I was the naïve one here on several counts, and that beat me down a little bit more.

This experience had made me a better trainer. Leading up to this, I had studied training methods, kinesiology, learnt the names of muscle groups in Latin, I had GNVQs and certifications for advanced fitness instruction, and had taken and passed many practical and theoretical tests on fitness, exercise, and nutrition. Nevertheless, I was not taught some of the basic factors that would actually make the difference for some of my clients – "Mind-set and what to expect when starting out."

It struck me that my personal experience in fitness and exercise counted for a lot more than my education, and this gave extra value to my clients. Although, it still took me a while to figure out how to best approach the situation of mind-set in a potential client such as this one.

So, how do you work on getting the correct mind-set? I have explained this in great detail in my book *Fitness & Exercise Motivation*; and if you are interested in motivation and mind-set training to further solidify your efforts, I would strongly suggest that you start right there before even thinking about exercise routines. My opinion that working on the mind is more important in most cases than training the body has already been addressed in this book. Thus, hopefully, this has reinforced my thoughts further, and this true account above serves as a good echo.

The primary idea that you should take away from this point is that you should prepare yourself for a long bumpy journey that will challenge you. But, at the end of the journey, it will all be worth it.
I can tell you that achieving your fitness goals will enrich your whole life. It will not only make you healthy and strong physically, but it will greatly improve your mental strength and your self-worth.
If you can appreciate that it will be challenging, that it will take time, and that it will be a mental struggle as well as physical one, you will have a head start over most others.

#2 - Not having a plan

Another common mistake is not having a plan. This is another big one that can slowly haemorrhage any motivation and aspiration that has collected. When one decides to get started with health and fitness, it is either the result of many years of knowing that they should, saying that they will do so soon, or both. They will have enough motivation to work out at a gym, go for a run, or decide to cook a healthy meal – and that is great!
However, one impromptu gym session or run won't make any difference, and a single healthy meal every now and again isn't going to change a whole lot. So, if the training sessions and meals are sporadic, and there is no structure or plans of progression, there is going to be minimal to zero results. The worst thing about this, and it is the part that I hate to see the most, is that the all-important motivation, which should have been the catalyst to life-changing effects, is entirely depleted. And, if you lose this in the early stages, it's harder to get back.

However, if you have a solid plan in place before you start, which —

- looks ahead at least six weeks
- is progressive
- suits your current fitness level
- has a nutritional program that relates to physical training

you are less likely to lose your motivation in the early stages and are far more likely to get your results as quickly as possible. You will also stick to your plans with the aid of you continued motivation until you actually see your first real results. At this point, your motivation will be boosted.

Planning is a very important part, and again, it is overlooked by most; even by guys who are in shape and have been regular gymgoers for a while. This situation, however, is slightly different, and the main problem here is the lack of progression. But, this is still related to not having a progressive plan in place that will best get the chosen result. It doesn't stop at having a good plan though; you still need to execute it correctly, which leads us on nicely to the next big mistake.

#3 Going Through The Motions

As well as training people on a personal level, I often used to instruct the odd exercise class collectively. It was really enjoyable to conduct circuit training classes and come up with new ideas for the group of regulars who joined in. It was here that I first noticed a trait in people that I had previously overlooked, and from then on, I began to see it everywhere. I began to see it more and more in the classes that I taught, in people training on their own, in people who had training partners; I even tested this out on my personal training clients, and I must admit that there were, and still are, times when I have had to remind myself of this inbuilt trait that we all appear to have in my own training sessions.
As the circuit class that I used to run was comprised of people with a fairly wide range of ability, during these sessions I would often give two variations of an exercise for a target muscle group – one for less

able-bodied people or beginners and one for the more advanced guys. When the circuit training was underweight, I found myself constantly having to tell people that they should be doing the more challenging of these exercise variations.

It still surprises me today how many people will join a gym, develop a strong and regular visiting habit (Arguably one of the toughest pieces of the puzzle), but will not achieve any results. One of the main reasons for this is that they will only go through the motions of the training and not challenge themselves sufficiently during the actual workouts.

Visiting the gym or doing regular exercise is one thing, but if you are taking the time and effort to be there or do the exercises, why not take the most out of it? The simple truth here is that if you aren't challenging yourself enough, your physical results will reflect this. My theory is that if you spend forty-five minutes or an hour in the gym or on an exercise session, you may as well make it count by pushing yourself and "getting your money's worth" rather than just using the exercise sessions as a way of self-justification alone.

Beginners are vulnerable to give in to this attitude. It is also probably set in the midst of the fight or flight instinct of humans.. If you don't need to expend all of this energy and make yourself uncomfortable, it's best not to do it at all.

However, the reality is that we don't spend endless days tracking our dangerous meals through harsh environments anymore. We are (on land at least) at the top of the food chain. We also have easy access to everything. This is why we need exercise routines that are physically challenging; we need ways apart from chasing woolly mammoths, wrestling wild boars, or climbing trees to harvest fruit to keep our bodies functional, strong, and efficient.

Therefore, the next time you train, ask yourself –

"Is this as challenging as fighting off a pack of wolves or spending time harvesting a large area of crops by hand?"

Or, if you would rather look at it in a less philosophical and imaginative way –

28

"Am I really getting the most out of this training session, or am I just going through the motions? Could I honestly say that this is challenging me enough?"

#4 Lack Of Self teaching

Learning how something works will help you better understand it, and with this knowledge, you can make it function more efficiently. If someone sat me down in front of a PC and said, "Jim, open up Word and write a letter thanking all of the readers or listeners of the audio version of your books for their purchases and congratulate them on their future fitness success." I would know exactly what to do and how best to do it. It's probably right to say that most people would know exactly what to do here too.

However you have learnt to do this, whether it was from a class that you had attended or whether it was a requirement of your working life, this kind of thing is common knowledge, and it was probably due to a necessity that you had learnt that skill.

Unfortunately, learning correct nutrition, developing positive mental health, and learning to exercise correctly are not seen as necessities, and if you didn't take a personal interest in these subjects, there is no real reason for you to need them.

This is why it is so important to self-teach. Since you are reading or listening to this, I would imagine that you are already of this ilk; so, there is no need to over-articulate this point. Nevertheless, I would like to express a few opinions.

If you are already into self-teaching, that's great; I am too, but one of the things that I would be aware of, especially in the fitness industry, is that there are many different ways of training, and every fitness professional will have differing opinions to a certain extent. Thus, it can get very confusing, very quickly. This is why I believe that the most useful and effective use of your time is not to look at our "great and ultimate training routines" or "ground-breaking new training systems" or the "ultimate all-in-one super weight-loss diet", but to first understand the functions of the human body.

Learn and understand –

- cardio vascular and resistance exercise functions
- the five food groups and recommended amounts
- muscle functions and which bodily movements utilise which muscles (basic kinesiology)
- the relation between body fat percentage, exercise volume, and calorie intake

As you probably know, this is all basic stuff, but in my experience, this knowledge is rarely understood to a standard that trainers and would-be fitness and weight-loss success stories should possess. Once you understand these basics, you can go ahead and start building on them. You will also develop the means to make a clear judgement on whether a particular method of training will suit you and your plans.

I am a big advocate of self-teaching, but I am also an equally big advocate of KISS – Keep It Simple Stupid. This leads us on to the last big mistake.

#5 Making it too complicated (focusing too much on theory)

There are literally hundreds of ways that you can train to get a similar fitness and weight-loss result. Although some training methods may be more efficient than others, the exercise choices of one method may be more fun for certain individuals than others, or the frequency of training sessions might suit certain people better than others. It all comes down to one basic rule –

"You do the work, you get the results."

If you take too long to find a new and innovative training routine or frequently try finding faults in potential fitness plans, you will never truly get started or stick to a regime long enough to see results; there will always be a newer and better regime that you would come across.

While it is important to self-teach, and while it is very beneficial to understand the science behind training, nutrition, and physiology, your focus should actually be on continuing training sessions and making sure that you stay consistent with your diet. It is the practical activities you do that will yield physical result, and the physical result is your ultimate goal.

Let's say, for instance, that Billy needs to lose a lot of weight. He's forty years old and has never been interested in fitness all his life until now, when it has become a necessity. He has heard that walking a mile every day will help him a lot; so, he goes to google and looks for "weight-loss success stories from walking". This search shows a ton of before and after pictures, another ton of weight-loss supplements, and yet another ton of fitness clothing. Before going for his first walk, Billy decides that he needs the right footwear; so, he orders some of the most popular running shoes of his size. Two days later, these are delivered to him; they fit very nicely and are very comfortable with a nice cushioned shock absorbing sole. With his brand new running shoes, Billy decides that he needs to learn about beginner fitness and running before he finally goes for his first fat burning walk. So, it's off to YouTube! While he's down this YouTube rabbit hole, Billy zeroes in on a theory that bare foot is far better for your knees, posture, overall fitness, and it will help to keep you injury-free. This is quite the revelation to Billy, so he decides that barefoot may be the way that he should do his fitness walks. However, as he is new to fitness, he decides that he needs to lose his initial weight first by doing a different form of cardio; so, he goes back to google to look for information on "Weight -oss success stories from exercise bike". The process starts all over again.

If Billy had just decided to put on his regular footwear and walk a mile on day one, he would have completed his first cardio session. If there were any problems with his feet caused by his footwear, he could have then bought a pair of running shoes right away, ready for his next session; or, if the problem wasn't too bad, ordered them and made do with his original shoes until they were delivered. This way Billy would have had three miles of fat burning to his name before he gave up on the idea in favour of another training method due to the overload of conflicting information that made him overcomplicate his plans.

This is just a quick and simple example of how fitness goals can be entirely blocked by overcomplicating your plans, and there are countless ways how this could happen. For instance, people do the same thing with diet and nutrition, or even sports specific fitness goals like building muscle or developing endurance.

"So, do I self-teach or don't? C'mon Jim, you sound like a back peddling politician!" I hear you say.

The more you learn and the more fitness knowledge you acquire, the better equipped and more efficient you will be when it comes to earning physical fitness results; there is absolutely no doubt about that. However, this takes time, and as with most scientific and theory-based work, you can't know the outcome of something unless you have data from practical experiments to observe from. There are plenty of starting points and training templates to choose from; several of my other books are dedicated to this. So, choose one, start the training, and address any hurdle that you encounter when you encounter it. In my opinion, this approach is far more valuable than theorising and deliberating. With long-term fitness and weight-loss, there are no two identical journeys, and everyone will have a different challenge; you are the pioneer of your own success.

Learning is important, but getting started is more important. Learning as you go along and making subtle changes when you need them is the way to go.

To sum up this point in simple terms, when you decide to embark on a fitness journey, you should be aware of the potential for overcomplicating things, and the negative effect that this can have on your plans. So, if you find yourself putting off a physical training session or delaying your entire fitness journey due to theory and research, it will help to refer back to this list:

- Remember – for physical results – any level of physical activity is better than just sitting down and researching.
- Learning is important, but getting started is more important.
- Pick a basic plan and stick to it. If you need to change things, make small changes rather than big ones.
- Don't sacrifice your physical efforts and activities for theory.
- Drip-feeding information and learning as you go is all part of a sustainable, progressive journey to fitness and weight-loss success.

SIX

PYRAMIDS OF CHANGE

For the purpose of this book, we will focus on three types of fitness tips that you can follow. Each one of these is important for development and progress in any type of fitness venture. Everyone is different, and a challenge to one may be less of a challenge to another, which means that a mental challenge may be easier for me to overcome than you, but a diet challenge may be easier for you to overcome than me. So, I would need to make the changes that relate to diet a priority, whereas you would need to make the changes that relate to mind-set a priority. Nonetheless, all three categories of change will ultimately connect nicely with each other and work to form a great synergy that will become the major fundamentals of your fitness or weight-loss success story.

Treat these categories as a three-layered pyramid-shaped jigsaw puzzle – you can't complete the puzzle without all three pieces. Mind-set is at the base, diet in the middle, and exercise at the apex.

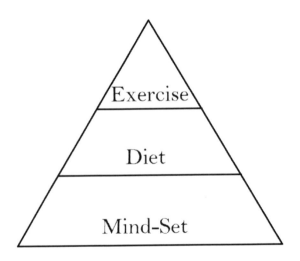

The three categories of change are the following:

- Mind-set
- Diet
- Exercise

Mind-set

In my opinion, this is where it all starts. If you have never been able to achieve sustainable fitness or weight-loss results before, but you have always dreamt of the success that could be yours, this should be your starting point. It is completely understandable that someone who has never taken an interest in fitness, weight-loss, or dieting before, but wishes to start now, would look at exercise or diet as their first port of call. If you are in this boat, you should definitely start here.

It is the mental robustness that comes from consistent, constructive development of your mental health that will help you make the right dietary decisions, keep you on track with your exercise choices, and keep you in the game long enough for you to create solid, positive habits that will finally change your life.

Therefore, if you have neglected your positive mental health development in the past or started diets and exercise plans that got you nowhere, before you make the same mistakes again, before you even think about changing your diet, lifting a set of dumbbells, or going for a jog, you should sit down and put in some work on developing the driving force for your physical fitness success – you should start training your mind.

Diet

Small tweaks and changes in your diet can have drastic effects on your body composition, not to mention your general health and state of mind. The diet changes that we will look at later in the book will vary from seemingly insignificant to a bit more time-consuming and inconvenient. However, please remember that any change can be very hard; then again, the longer you stick with it, the easier it will become to stick to until it becomes your second nature and a part of who you are.

Diet is a big one. With a change in diet alone and minimal to zero exercise, you can achieve some outstanding weight-loss goals. As mentioned before, this is a favourite starting point among the beginners since it seems to be a straightforward and fairly hassle-free entry into the weight-loss game. However, if the changes are too drastic or too much, too soon, and too inconvenient, and if you lack knowledge of good nutrition, the diet plans will be unsustainable and won't last long.

So, the diet category should not be taken lightly, and in the vast majority of cases, it should be the second focus of change and tweaks after mind-set.

Exercise

Starting an exercise regimen, going for a run, or lifting a few weights is as common a starting point as diet for a lot of people. However, as I have explained in many of my other books, blog posts, social media posts, and even directly to people's faces, "Exercise is only the icing on the cake, and without the mind-set and diet, you are unlikely to achieve the fitness results that you really want."

If you have managed to read this far into the book, you will know how important these other ingredients are to this philosophy. I would be devastated to hear that if you have always struggled with fitness and weight-loss, you will now go on to make the mistake of spending your time looking at exercise routines rather than the first building block that is mind-set.

Yes! Exercise is important, but without the mind-set to drive you along and the correct nutrition to fuel you, your journey will be short-lived.

Although the top of the pyramid, which represents exercise, appears to be a complete pyramid by itself, you and I know that when it's in the same picture as the foundations it was meant to stand upon, it has a place of its own on top; and when they are placed together, neither piece looks unfinished.

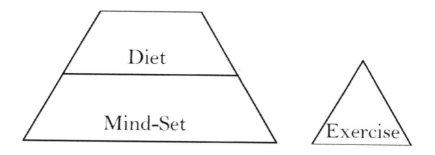

Are you ready to change? And are you ready to start working towards your fitness and weight-loss goals?

If you can answer these questions with a resounding "Yes", then you are ready to get started; but, if you can't, you still have some more reading or re-reading to do before you start making your changes.

- Are you willing to be open-minded and move out of your comfort zone if need be?
- Are you ready to commit to your fitness goal for the foreseeable future?
- Do you understand that this will take time and that you *will* face challenges, even if the a change that you make appears to be very small?
- Do you understand that this is a long process, and if you stay consistent, you'll be forging a healthier life for yourself?

Okay, so if you are really ready to start changing things, let's get cracking! I really look forward to the start of someone's fitness endeavour; this is because I know how good it feels when you actually see your work starting to pay off, someone comments on how good you are looking, or how well you are doing. This is the point of no return for most people, as there is nothing quite like this feeling of accomplishment. This feeling is amplified for those who have struggled the most or have come from notable obesity or significant mental health conditions, such as depression, stress, or anxiety.

Personally, this kind of success impresses me as much as the gold medal winners in the Olympics. I have as much respect for people who come from dire health and fitness conditions or extreme cases of depression and other mental health issues to earn their fitness success as I have for those gold medal winners.

SEVEN

A DIFFERENT PATH

In the next section, I will list the twenty-five fitness tips that I would implement in my life in the order that I would implement them if I was to start from scratch.

To better understand my angle and portray it with more clarity, I will build up a fictional profile and character that could have easily been me if my life had played out along a different path.

Its May 23rd, I'm thirty-five years old, my height is 5'9", and I weigh 230lbs.

I have an office job that takes up most of my time. I am comfortable there, but after a hard day at work, it's nice to come home and watch the TV with some convenient tasty food. I love my food, so I eat what I want, when I want.

PC games are a big part of my life. I have a great gaming set-up that can keep me immersed in it for hours. On the weekends, when there are no work commitments, I can stock up on snacks and pizza and get absorbed into my favourite MMORPG.

I go out for a few drinks every now and again with my colleagues, but I don't really socialise that much.

I have wanted to lose some of the weight that has been creeping up on me over the years for a while, but it has come to the point where I have realised that unless I change some things about my lifestyle, my weight will continue to increase, and my health will really start to suffer.

I often feel depressed about my situation and wish that there was a button that would just get me out of it and give me another shot; but, there isn't... Wait! What's this on Amazon? *Health & Fitness Tips That Will Change Your Life*

There's always a light at the end of the tunnel, but in all seriousness, there are only a few differences from the Jim that I am in this reality and the Jim that I would be in the fictional reality that I just described.

The Jim that is actually writing this book loves his food, loves his PC games, likes to socialise, especially when there are a few drinks involved; he is thirty five years old, 5'9" tall, and he has a desk job.

However, he also knows what it takes to lead a healthy lifestyle. He has learnt to appreciate the value of sustained fitness and healthy eating efforts. He has self-funded his official fitness education and self-taught through his own fitness efforts; he has learnt more lessons on his personal fitness journey than you might think, and these lessons have proven to be invaluable, not only for him but for all the people that read his work and take his advice.

The fictional Jim does, however, have a far better gaming PC and set-up, but the Jim that is writing this book is working on that one.

Somehow, if these realities merged, and the brain of the Jim writing this book was transplanted to the body and fictional reality of the other Jim, what would he do? Or, more accurately – what would I do?

First, I would probably admire the far superior gaming set up that I now had; but soon after, I would start to plan my rise to fitness success.

As this new body of mine has been used to eating what it wanted, when it wanted, I would have a hard time with a straight switch from the diet that the body had been on to the diet of the Jim that had just taken over. Of course, it would be possible to act with extreme resolve and start eating a healthy fat-burning diet, start training five times a week, and become a health and fitness saint overnight; but, for most people, as outlined in an earlier chapter, change is hard; and the more extreme the change, the more uncomfortable and challenging the whole thing will be. Moreover, we all know the danger of too much, too soon.

This is why I would plan my changes, and I would plan to make one change every two weeks. Due to the lack of physical activity, quality nutrition, and a general lack of interest in healthy living that my new body has been subjected to over the years, I would start with a small change every two weeks.

Since there has been no structure or routine in the way of health and fitness, if too much of a burden is placed on the body, and if there is too much stress, I may be in danger of the body taking over the mind of the Jim that is here to fix it. So, a small change every two weeks should keep me motivated and hungry for the next change. Two weeks is a fairly long time to keep up a habit; and, it is said that it only takes four weeks to make a habit stick; if this is true, I would be halfway towards making my change or good habit stick at the point of starting my next change or tweak. This is how the whole process is compounded.

It all starts off at a slow pace, but as the weeks and months pass by, the fitness tips that you have followed or the changes that you have made persist and compound to create the effect of a growing snowball that's rolling down a snow covered mountain – it gets bigger and bigger until it is unstoppable. In this case, the big unstoppable snowball will be in the form of fitness and fat loss results. However, before you have an unstoppable snowball, you have to make a small one with your hands; roll it around in the new snow until its big enough to use its own weight as momentum, before you set it on its journey to exponential growth.

In the pages that follow, I will list the twenty-five tweaks, fitness tips, or habits, whatever you want to call them and give my reasons for making the change. Of course, this will be based on the fictional profile and situation that we just heard about. Although this is a fictional character, I have addressed some common issues that a lot of people, men and women, can relate to – comfort zones causing stagnation, thirty-somethings who get a realisation, lack of nutritional understanding, feelings of depression, the modern push-button-for-results attitude, etc. Nonetheless, I have also tried to keep the fiction close to home and not stray too far from my own lifestyle; for example, the fictional Jim does not have any children. This would add a whole new dynamic to the order of fitness tips or changes to follow and probably the entirety of the list. I do not have any experience with raising children, so I would only be guessing at how I would fit things in around them. In this case, my advice may be impractical.

41

Yes, every time someone with young children reads the last few sentences or hears it on the audio version, I get hit with "mind bullets" that take the form of a familiar statement with words to the effect of, "Yes, it's so much easier without kids. If I was in your shoes, I'd do this easy!"

I understand that some people have children and they can be a handful; some work jobs with unsocial hours; some people are physically impaired, and some don't have access to a gym. The list can go on.

There is a great chapter in my other book, *Fitness & Exercise motivation* that runs into detail about this natural response; and believe me, I have said similar things about others who I have observed excelling in sports, bodybuilding, and promotions at work. The bottom line here is that everyone has their own set of challenges to overcome, and as I heard Jim Rhone say once,

"The same wind blows on us all"

Sure, there may be some things that are out of your control, but if you can sit back and with true, assured honesty say, "Yes, I have done my absolute best", then you will get to where you want to be.

EIGHT

MY 25 FITNESS TIPS

I didn't just pick the number twenty-five out of the air. As with all of my guides, there is a theory behind this madness. If I chose to plan twenty-five changes to drastically improve this lifestyle, if I do well on these changes and implement a single change every two weeks, I will have effectively planned out a full year of progression.

A year may appear daunting to a lot of people, but it really need not. Most people I personally know or have known who have expressed a desire to bring positive changes to their bodies in the past are still expressing the same longing several years later. I will admit that this gets me down and frustrates me more than just a little. I would have loved to see them take my advice several years ago and reap the second, third, or even fourth harvest of their new lifestyle; but often times, they are not ready to start.

Hopefully, we are. Don't be the guy or gal that puts it off; don't be the one who says, "maybe tomorrow." Before you know it, tomorrow will be next year, and you will have missed out on some fantastic life-changing opportunities.

This is my list of twenty five fitness tips and changes made over the span of a year based on fictional Jim mentioned in the previous chapter.

Feel free to emulate these fitness tips exactly, but I would advise that you tailor your changes to suit your own personal circumstances.

Fitness Tip #1 (Mind-set) – On the first week and at the start of it all, I would be positive – I would write down or make a mental note of at least one positive thing that happened to me in the day for every day of the week.

Why?

I have reiterated this often, but it is worth saying once again. Working on developing a positive mental attitude will be invaluable when it comes to facing some of the challenges that lie ahead. By actively looking for positivity in your day to day life and making this a regular habit, your positivity will become passive, and this will help to build your mental strength. Everybody endures days that drag them down when nothing seems to go right; but as I demonstrated earlier, there is always a light in the dark. You simply have to recognise it. If you are late for work, get into an argument with a loved one, fall off a ladder, or even get hit by a car, if you can get up, you can look for that light.

Changing your attitude from glass half empty to glass half full may take a while; Therefore, it's imperative to get this aspect of your health and fitness journey started as soon as possible. This component of your mind-set development will be of major value to your efforts and positively impact your character.

Fitness Tip #2 (Diet) – My second change would be to start drinking at least 2 litres of water every day.

Why?

Being hydrated correctly doesn't mean that you are not thirsty. Look at it this way – Water is the vehicle that transports nutrients from the food that you eat around your body. So, if you are correctly hydrated, your body will altogether be more efficient. You will be more alert; you will have more energy; your muscles will function better; you will have fewer toxins in your body, and the list goes on. Moreover, if you are going to start eating healthier and work out from this point onwards, it makes sense to get used to drinking plenty of water early on in the process so that you get the most out of your new diet choices and exercise sessions.

I know from personal experience that if I turn up at the gym ready to hit my workout, and I am not sufficiently hydrated, I struggle with the workout. Not only do I struggle with my usual weight on the bar, but I also struggle with the number of reps that I aim for. I feel lethargic and generally have a bad workout.

Taking your water intake seriously is a must. Not only does it help transport healthy nutrients around your body and makes it more efficient, but there are countless other benefits that are essential for fitness and health development that will aid you in your success.

Fitness Tip #3 (Exercise) – Four weeks into the regimen, as the next change, I would go for a walk every working day.

Why?

This would be my first change that involves exercise. There are many great reasons for choosing walking as my introductory exercise choice, but here are a few of the highlights that that demonstrate why this would be my first choice, given my specific situation. On the practical side of things, walking requires no equipment. It's easy to do; I don't need a gym membership; and I can do it at any time. However, I would also benefit from making this activity a part of my daily routine; this would ultimately become a solid foundation for transferable value. Believe it or not, the calories that I would be burning on my daily walk, the positive effects that it would have on my metabolism, and all of the other health benefits that are associated with walking would be the tip of the iceberg. I believe that its primary value would be the development of routine. Making regular exercise a part of daily life is one of the fundamentals of fitness progression. Therefore, acquiring this habit early on is very wise.

For the walking sessions themselves, I would aim for a continuous brisk walk for at least thirty minutes every day before breakfast. If you are looking for fat loss in particular, I have found that steady and regular cardio sessions are most effective at this stage and performing this exercise on an empty stomach, though it's essential, is a big added bonus. If you do decide to try cardio on an empty stomach, I would highly recommend that you eat a healthy breakfast to replenish you immediately after your session. You can consider eating a piece of fruit and a simple protein and carbs drink to refuel. There' more on eating later.

Fitness Tip #4 (Mind-set) – The next change that I would make would be to add some motivational material to my life. You could find time to read or listen to someone else's fitness success stories from books, audio books, or podcasts. Set aside a small amount of time every week; 10 mins, maybe 20 mins, or even an hour if you have it.

Why?

Getting up earlier than I usually do and going for a walk might sound easy, but I know that there will be days, especially in the early stages of this transformation, when I will struggle. Maybe it'll rain outside, it's going to be dark, and I would have had a late night playing on my awesome PC gaming set up. But, this is where it counts. I know for a fact from my experience as the other Jim that once I'm up and out, I would be so glad that I didn't "give it a miss today". Rest assured, there will be a time when one day off really won't make a difference, but that's way down the road. At the early stages, you need to be 100% committed.

To remind me of this, I may set the background of my phone to show a motivational quote that connects with me and reminds me of why I'm doing this; something to tell me, "Get your sorry ass out there". I'd have it on my phone because I use my phone as an alarm clock. To stop the alarm, I'd have no choice but to look right at it.

Fitness Tip #5 (Diet) – I would make a conscious effort to eat smaller portions at every meal.

Why?

This may be an obvious one, but it's a solid one. There are far more complex reasons, but in the interest of keeping this as free as possible of science and jargon, here is a simple explanation: Your body can only absorb a certain amount of nutrients in one go; so, if you are giving it more than it can handle on a regular basis, the excess nutrition will be stored as fat. If you are also cutting down on your portion sizes at every meal, you will be able to add more meals throughout the day. Developing a habit of eating "little and often" will earn you some other health and fat loss boons that some people rely on as their main focus for weight-loss. Eating small amounts of healthy, nutritious food every two to three hours will give your metabolism a massive boost. If you do this long enough, your body will become accustomed to this pattern. It will become very efficient at its job, and your metabolism will work to minimise fat storage.

This is our metabolism in the simplest terms, and it is important to remember that regular exercise is a huge part of helping your metabolism become more efficient.

If you decide to follow this fitness tip, here is one more little gem to further consider: If you are struggling with hunger after you eat, it may be because you are eating too fast. If you take your time with your food, you are less likely to be hungry when you finish. It is said that it takes a while for your brain to receive the "I'm full, stop eating" signal after you are actually full. So, with this in mind, you should have an easier time if you eat your meals slower than usual. If you are eating with a knife and fork, try putting them on the table between bites while you chew. Also, try chewing longer. You may be surprised at how effective this is.

Fitness Tip #6 (Exercise) – Learn a new resistance exercise movement that can be performed at home (bodyweight squat is a great first choice). I would do 3 sets of 10–15 reps of this exercise immediately before my walking sessions. I would also go on to add a new exercise choice every two weeks until I am doing 8–10 exercise movements immediately before my cardio at 10-15 reps of each.

Why?

Most beginners who are looking to lose some body fat and get in shape without exercise movements fall back on cardio exercise since it feels right to go for a run in order to get the best results. In fact, cardiovascular exercises are only a part of the puzzle. Resistance training will tone muscles, and many can also be used to burn fat. Nevertheless, the most efficient and quickest way to burn fat is to utilise both forms of exercise. This is how I always convince people who are averse to the idea of bodyweight exercises, using exercise bands, or lifting dumbbells: "Think of your muscles as your on-board fat burning machines. Your muscles want to use your fat deposits to get stronger, but you have to give them an appetite before they will work for you; so, by challenging them, you are making them hungry! The more lean muscle that you have, the more fat you will burn in your workouts."

Again, this is a simple way of looking at a complex biological process, albeit with a few added quirks; but the idea behind it holds up.

Why resistance before cardio? This is again linked to your metabolism. If you go out and do a thirty minute jog, walk, or run from cold, great! You will have completed your exercise, and the benefits will show in due course if you keep it up. However, it takes around ten minutes for your body and metabolism to start functioning at its most efficient, in this case, fat burning. This means that during a thirty minute cardio session alone, we will only get about twenty minutes of good fat burning in. If you train with resistance exercises immediately before you go for your cardio session, your body will already be in its zone and work to burn calories more efficiently. This means that we would achieve more efficient fat burning from our cardio sessions.

As the weeks progress, you would be adding more resistance movements, and eventually, you would be incorporating all of your major muscle groups into your resistance workout.

If you exactly follow all of these fitness tips, you may already be doing fasted cardio. If this is the case, I would advise that you switch to eating your breakfast before training when you start to incorporate your third exercise choice. The reason for this is that your body needs fuel to perform; the benefits of fasted cardio would simply be outweighed by the benefits of resistance exercise and its subsequent increased intensity in general. Lack of fuel in your system may start to hinder your progress at this point.

Fitness Tip #7 (mind-set) – Next, I would post my progress and plans on my social media networks. I would probably add a picture or two as well. From now on, I would update this every week with my progress and add the details of the change that I planned to make on the night before I actually make it. I would post once every week on the same day and at the same time.

Why?

In this day and age, the social media has become common in a lot of people's lives. I don't see social media as a place for cat videos, sneezing pandas, games, or pouting selfies (Although if someone points a camera at me, my face will instantly crease into an ironic pout or a ridiculous comic expression). I see social media channels as a way of putting information out there that could help others or my own self. If you decide to make a post telling people that you are going to do something, you will be held accountable for it, and this is a good thing. It is quite common for people who are new to fitness and weight-loss to want to keep their plans to themselves. This is because if they didn't make it or in their eyes, failed, they wouldn't have to explain to others why they stopped. With some of this extra accountability, the option of failing becomes far less of an option, and in some cases, it becomes non-existent. There are many other benefits of telling folks about your plans rather than accountability alone. You will more than likely have your close friends, family, and acquaintances contact you and encourage you to do well; you may even inspire others to follow in your footsteps, and the longer you post and the more you progress, you will find that you are building a support network that consists of lots of people rooting for you and wanting you to succeed. This also gives you a great chance to prove sceptics wrong.

Creating accountability is a smart thing to do, and it can be very powerful too. Yes, it can be hard to put yourself out there, make your plans public knowledge, and tell everyone what you are doing; but, if you had an opportunity to take the possibility of failure out of the equation, wouldn't you take it?

Fitness Tip #8 (Diet) – I will have a healthy breakfast every day; make this a "must do".

Why?

Most people have heard the expression "Breakfast is the most important meal of the day", and that's because it is actually very important. There are so many reasons that you should eat a good healthy breakfast. Not only will a healthy nutritious breakfast give you more energy throughout the day, it will also help you out so much more with your fitness, weight-loss, and lifestyle in general.

We have touched on the subject of metabolism and how understanding the basics of this will help you become more efficient at burning extra calories and ultimately help you lose your unwanted weight quicker in combination with resistance exercise and cardio. As surprising as it may sound, eating food actually helps with this too.

When you eat, your body has to work on processing the food that you give it. Believe it or not, this takes energy and actually uses calories to do so. If your body has been dormant (you have been sleeping) for several hours, your metabolism will slow down. If you eat first thing in the morning, your body will have to get to work on processing the food that you give it right away and get it ready for the day. Obviously, the higher the nutritional value of the food that you eat for your breakfast, the better.

Thus, eating a good breakfast kick-starts your body and your metabolism to make it start functioning right away. As a result, you will have more energy throughout the day. Another advantage of eating breakfast is that you are less likely to make bad food choices later on. For example, if you have missed breakfast, you may be enticed to eat donuts in the break room or unhealthy vending machine snacks at work. This is obviously not good for anyone following this plan. If this occurs, you will have failed to initiate your metabolism early on, and when it does commence after its long slumber, it has terrible fuel to work with. It will remain sluggish and not work with you and your weight-loss goals.

I know so many people who skip breakfast, and many of them are overweight. The common excuse is that they don't have enough time in the morning to eat breakfast. There should always be enough time to eat breakfast. Remember that it is "the most important meal of the day"; and so, it is important to make time for it. If you are not used to eating a healthy breakfast, it may take a few weeks to get your routine sorted, but that's exactly what this whole book is all about. There are a lot of options for healthy breakfasts; here is an example of a quick, nutritious, and balanced breakfast that will suit someone who is following a regular exercise routine –

1. Grab a bowl
2. Add ½ a cup of rolled oats, a scoop of whey protein (vanilla or chocolate works well), and a spoonful of natural peanut butter to the bowl
3. Fill a kettle with water and start heating it. Stop it before it has boiled so that the water is hot/warm but not boiling
4. Pour a little hot/warm water into the bowl and mix
5. Add some fresh blueberries
6. Get it in you

I eat this regularly. It's a really quick, easy, and all round good choice for breakfast meal, and it tastes great too.

Fitness Tip #9 (Mind-set) – This is a one-off, but it is still an action that I would take at this point – Sixteen weeks into the plan, I would revisit my reasons for starting my fitness journey.

Why?

At this point in any fitness or weight-loss journey, motivation might be low since the initial results may have slowed down or plateaued. This is quite normal. Since the future fitness tips will be followed, there will be more motivation and results heading your way. It is a critical time, and you need to work through it. This is actually the end point for many people; so, don't be one of them.

To guard against this, I'd get a new piece of motivational material. In my case, I would opt for a picture. This would be put up on my gaming desk, and it would be of Arnold when he was at his prime bodybuilding state back in the 80s. Arnold was an inspiration for the original Jim, so he can be here for his fictional out of shape counterpart. I'd take some time and have some fun personalising this picture, maybe by making the picture have a speech bubble on it with one of his quotes such as –

"If you don't find the time, if you don't do the work, you won't get the results."

This way, I would see my motivation every time I sit at my gaming desk, and if I hadn't done my training, neglected my diet, or passed up one of my new habits to play PC games, Arnold would be there, in my face, to put me straight.

It really won't take up much of your time. This may seem like an easy thing to do, but it will certainly be worth the effort. Not only will it take a few minutes to implement, it will also give you a boost in motivation. This is something that you can do at any point when you feel your motivation is diminishing. It's always a good idea to revisit and refresh your motivational material from time to time.

At this point in the whole process, there will have been a few big changes that have taken place; some will be more challenging than others, so having an easy one-off fitness tip to follow now will help you to take stock and make sure that all of the previous fitness tips that you have followed are still being practiced. It is, however, still important to make sure that you actually plan a change since this will keep you in the routine.

Fitness Tip #10 (Diet) – I would learn to cook a new healthy meal every week. I have to eat; so, why not have one night every week as my "experiment night".

Why?

Knowing the difference between bad and good food, and knowing the nutritional value and its function is one thing, but knowing how to create good meals from good food is an entirely new skill.

If you love food like I do, then why not learn how to create your own healthy meals? Learning to cook healthy food is such a valuable skill. If you have knowledge of seven to ten healthy recipes, you will never be at a loss for ideas when it comes to meal choices, and the more things you try, the better you will become at cooking. Eventually, you will have the confidence to experiment with different ingredients and even come up with your own healthy recipes.

If I had never cooked or didn't have knowledge of cooking clean, healthy, and nutritious food before, this is what I would do –

I would make a list of foods and things that I enjoy eating, not taking into account whether these foods were good or bad for me. I would then pick one from the list; let's say, for example, cheeseburgers. I would then look it up in a search engine and add one of the following words to it: healthy, Low-fat, low-sugar, Fat-burning. If you've not looked for healthy recipes like this before, you will be surprised at the ideas you will find.

If you haven't got it already, I have another freebie for you. I've created seven healthy recipes that you can use right off the bat. You will see from the pictures that I make all of them myself in my own kitchen; and I regularly make these meals for myself and Mrs Jims Health And Muscle. Most of these are a spin on my favourite foods. So, I can eat burgers, meatloaf, chilli, pizza, and not feel guilty about it. Check it out if you need some inspiration:

https://jimshealthandmuscle.com/#download-recipe

It's a good idea to pick one night every week to try out a new recipe. This way, if you plan to make something, and it all goes horribly wrong, it'll only be one night that you have to deal with it. On the other hand, if your cooking experiment is a screaming success, you have a healthy recipe in the bank that you can use another time or even allocate an evening every week to cook this on. For instance, Monday nights could be your "Thai chicken curry night", or you could have "Green veg and chicken breast stir-Friday"... See what I did there?

This skill can be very valuable, and if you are not used to cooking or are daunted by it, or even if you don't like the idea of it, I can tell you that you will probably be surprised at the feeling of accomplishment that comes from your creations in the kitchen. Cooking good food can become a real passion; so, give it a go.

Fitness Tip #11 (Exercise) – The next change would be focused on my cardio exercises. I would make sure that I am doing full forty-five minutes on my brisk walk. If I haven't managed to get to forty-five minutes on these sessions, I would make this a priority. I would add 1 minute per day until I get there. I would also add in a thirty-second to one minute jog at the halfway point of my cardio sessions.

Why?

Forty-five minutes of steady state cardio is a solid time frame if you are doing these sessions regularly; so, I would make this my time frame cap. By adding one minute to my cardio sessions every day, it would be very easy to get to the cap; even quicker with two minutes per day. These are very small, incremental increases that seem negligible at the time, but these small additions to cardio sessions are a great way to progress from a psychological point of view. So, if the prospect of a brisk walk for forty-five minutes is daunting to you, try this for yourself.

While I am working towards this cardio time cap, I would also work on becoming more efficient at fat burning in the timeslot allocated for my cardio sessions. The first thing that I would do is to add a thirty-second to one minute jog to this brisk walk, and I would throw this in at the midpoint of my cardio routine. When introducing jogging or running for the first time to your brisk walk, the midpoint is a great starting point. This is because you will be warmed up sufficiently, and you will also have some way to go when you return to your normal pace.

This is actually the most basic form of interval training. What benefits does interval training have compared to steady state?

Well, it has some great benefits that will help you burn more fat on your cardio sessions. As soon as you increase your pace, your heart rate will increase with it, and your body will need more energy. This is where your metabolism gets to work and goes looking for it.

More energy expended means more calories burned. The spike in heart rate means a boost in metabolism; and a boost in metabolism means more efficient fat burning. Another bonus that comes from adding this jog or run at the midway point is that for a time after, and in some cases the rest of the cardio session, the added spike of cardio from the jog will increase the heart rate, which results in a more intense and valuable second half of the session.

Fitness Tip #12 (Mind-set) – For my next step, I would aim to add more motivational audio. At this point, I would replace the music or the radio that played in my car on my drive to work with motivational audio content.

Why?

Keeping up with all of these new fitness tips will be hard; whoever you are, your motivation will always be tested, and again, it will always be diminishing unless you keep on top of it, maintain its state, and strive to nurture its growth. This is a small change that won't add any stress, take any time, but it will help to keep you going. If you find the right motivational material to listen to, it may even completely relight the fire inside you and make an immense difference to your progress.

When you look for motivational audio material, you will find a broad spectrum to choose from. "General motivation" is a good start. Although if you can, you should try and identify what you respond to best. If you can pinpoint any specific areas of particular weakness that you have, this will be more valuable. You could search for motivational material that addresses your main weakness directly; and if you don't find anything that hits it on the head, just work back from there and settle for the closest match.

For example, the fictional Jim that exists in this book really struggles to get motivated to start his exercise sessions. Once he has started, it's okay; and when he has finished, he feels accomplishment. It's just getting ready and out of the door for his cardio training is what he really struggles with. Thus, Jim would go to his favourite online audio marketplace and use the search term "Fitness and Exercise motivation". I'm sure that he would find something to listen to that was written by a name that sounded familiar.

However, everyone has a different make-up and faces different personal challenges. You may find getting up and out for your exercise sessions easier than you had imagined at first, but you may struggle in other areas such as your diet or staying focused. So, you can search for motivational material that addresses these problems.

Do not underestimate a little fitness tip like this; it may seem insignificant, but motivation is the driving force that ultimately carries you to success. Therefore, the more attention and relevant material that you feed your motivation, the better it will be sustained, and any amount of repetition will help your cause.

Fitness Tip #13 (Diet) – I would do a three to five day detox for the next phase of diet changes using fresh fruits and vegetables and a juicer. This would be the start of using juice as part of my long-term diet.

Why?

Over the last few years, I have become a big fan of the health and nutritional benefits that juice offers. For me, juicing is one of the best, if not the best and most efficient delivery systems of quality nutrition that you can get, and it has become part of mine and Mrs Jims Health And Muscles daily routine.

I won't go into the many benefits of drinking juice made from fresh fruits and vegetables since there are lots, but I find that the best way to sum it up is to think along these lines:

- Everyone knows that greens are good for you, and with juicing, it's possible to get the nutrients from big handfuls of these "super greens" into your body in only a few gulps
- Because the nutrients are being extracted from the fibrous material of these superfoods, the nutrients get absorbed into your system significantly faster.

- If you have not juiced before, you would be surprised at the variety of fruits and vegetables that you can juice and mix together without the juice tasting as you would imagine.
- This type of nutrition is amazing for the functioning of your systems. With a body that processes food efficiently, you will burn more fat, you will be more energised, and juicing will help you get a wide range of nutrition from a lot of different fruit and vegetables at once. This nutrition will be absorbed into your body extremely well.

"Okay Jim, If juicing is so amazing, why have you not used it until now?"

I would love to say that juicing is quick and easy with no mess or inconvenience, but I would be a big liar if I told you that! I have been into health and fitness for many years; I have made many sacrifices and put myself through a lot of hardship and inconvenience to achieve my fitness goals in the past, but after all of this, there's yet to be a morning when I welcome my juicing experience. Even though I have managed to get a system in place that takes only ten minutes from start to finish if I don't mess around, I still feel that this is a big chore. Although looking at the facts, theories, and common sense about juicing – to prepare the fruit and vegetables, juice them, and then clean the juicer thoroughly before actually drinking the juice – I can't deny that the payoff is so great that the inconvenience of actually preparing the juice pale into insignificance. Its more than worth it.

I'm sure that if juicing was part of the change earlier on in mine or anyone else's journey, it would be considered too big of a modification and too much a hassle to be worth it. It may even shock the beginner into submission.

Although at this stage, the beginner – in this case fictional Jim – Will be ready to give this a try. Moreover, after the previous change, he may feel ready for a bigger challenge. As fictional Jim has been more conscious of diet and healthy eating in general, he will benefit a lot more at this point too. When his juice detox is over, moving forward, he will benefit far more. So, he will open the door at this point on the start of his juice adventure and step right into a juice detox.

A great introduction to juicing would be to go all out for a few days and start with a juice detox.

For a lot of people, a juice detox or any other kind of detox may be a quick way to lose a few pounds in a short time. In my opinion, this is a pointless exercise. Yes, if you do a juice detox for three to five days or longer, you will almost certainly lose a few pounds; but as soon as you finish the detox and carry on eating as you normally would, those extra pounds that you lost will come right back, and your efforts will have been for nothing.

For us, those extra few pounds that we lost on the detox are a by-product of our main aim and only really serve as a bonus. We are focused on the long-term effects and the progression of sustained change, and that's our main reason for doing a detox.

Once again, I will cut out all the jargon and biological science and speak in a layman's terms – by doing a juice detox, we will reset our digestive system or give it a service, replacing worn out parts with new ones. By doing this, when the juice detox is over, the healthy food that we are now eating will be even more useful for our bodies. Our metabolism will function more efficiently, and we will get even more value from our workouts. To top this off, we would also have a great insight into the world of juicing and maybe start to think about adding a juice into our daily diet at some point.

Drinking Juice made from fresh fruits and vegetables really is an efficient way to get these vital nutritious foods into our body, and I would highly recommend trying this out if you have not done it before. I will also reiterate that it can be time-consuming and messy, especially at first, but if you persevere and experiment, you will find a system that you can work with that is time efficient and fits in with your daily schedule.

A juice detox at this point with a view to a more long-term sustainable approach to regular juicing would be an excellent catalyst to your fitness progression. If your motivation or progression is slowing down, it will almost certainly serve to boost results and give it a new lease of life.

Fitness Tip #14 (Diet) – I would prepare my own fresh healthy lunch for work every day.

Why?

Although it may not sound so, this is another fairly big change to make. Prepping a tuna salad, chicken breast and brown pasta, or turkey and brown rice wholemeal burrito (some ideas for you) may not sound like a big deal, but if you are not accustomed to prepping your own meals for your day at work, this can cause you some problems. You may find that it will make you late for work. You may also come to prepare your food and not actually have the right ingredients; so you settle for vending machine snacks again. You may also simply not have any inspiration or ideas for food choices.

To make this a smooth change, its best to do a bit of planning beforehand. The first step that I would take is to research one idea that seems like a good choice. For example, tuna salad. This seems like it could be a healthy option.

If I was to work every weekday, I would need to make this meal five times; so, it's a great idea to make sure that you get enough ingredients stocked up to cover five tuna salads. For my tuna salad, I would -

1. Slice a good few handfuls of iceberg lettuce and put this into the bottom of a sealable container that would double up as my lunchbox
2. Chop some cherry tomatoes and throw them in too.
3. Slice about half of a sweet red pepper and add it to the salad
4. Add a small handful of cooked red kidney beans to the lunchbox
5. Chop a spring onion and add this to the lunchbox.
6. Drain a full tin of tuna. If you have the funds and extra time, you could also cook a fresh tuna steak. This would be placed on top of everything in the lunchbox.
7. Finish the whole thing off with a drizzle of balsamic vinaigrette and cracked black pepper.

I would make sure that I had enough of this ingredients to make five tuna salads for the week ahead of me.

Make sure that you have a solid container that you can use to carry your lunch in. I find that Tupperware tubs or something similar are your best bet; they are solid, they seal nicely, and you can wash them easily. Get one or two of these.

All you have to do now is work on your morning routine of throwing all this in together. Like everything else, this may take a bit of time to get used to at first, but if you stick at it, it will start to fit in to your routine.

If you struggle with time in the morning, this could be a part of your evening routine; make your salad and put it in the fridge ready for your next day at work.

At first, I would only choose one lunch option since adding five different meal preps to a new routine is going to add more pressure to the whole change. Each meal prep will require a different routine; so, it's best to get one routine finely tuned and working like a well-oiled machine before working on the next. The less effort and less variables in each change that you make, the better; the more efficient that you can be with your changes, the more changes that you can make, and the easier it will be to take on the next.

Fitness Tip #15 (Diet) – I would plan for six days of healthy evening meals.

Why?

If I had been adhering to my healthy cooking, self-taught lessons, I would have enough to start allocating each recipe to each evening bar one (I have plans for the seventh day, which will be revealed later).

Similar to the last change, I would need to do a bit of planning. The main thing that I would need to do is to make sure that I have enough ingredients stocked up to do well on these plans. On the day before I push the button for this change, I would visit the grocery store and buy all the ingredients for my next week of evening meals. For some people, this may be a lot to plan, and it might be that their evenings that are time restricted. If this is the case for you, it may be easier to take one day at a time and add a new healthy recipe to a new night each week until you have all six evening meals covered. Nevertheless, as mentioned in an earlier change, it might help you to take the attitude of "I have to eat, so I have to cook. I may as well cook this". The sooner you can get used to cooking these recipes and fitting them into your life, the sooner you will benefit from this more healthy diet and lifestyle.

Thus, every evening meal from now on will be good food that is healthy and nutritious. The food that I will be eating from now on will be of value to my body. This is a big leap in the right direction and is now of exponential value to my efforts.

Fitness Tip #16 (Diet) - Introduce my cheat night; its reward time!

Why?

Not all changes are challenging, and if you enjoy your food, you may feel that you have sacrificed an awful lot of enjoyment so far. Moreover, if this fitness endeavour is to be successful, it has to be sustainable. I am of the opinion that a good level of health, fitness, and weight management is only worth pursuing if it is for the long-term and a part of a lifestyle rather than a project with an end date.

If someone told me that if I wanted to lose weight, I would never again be able to set foot inside a pizzeria or that a juicy cheeseburger with fries and ketchup was never to pass my lips again or that I had to forget the taste of chocolate, cake, or ice-cream, I would seriously question whether it was worth it.

So, naughty foods that you love but would associate with unhealthy living, obesity, and general bad health are not totally off limits for the rest of your life. It all comes down to moderation. I have written about my own cheat night several times in my other books and on my blog before, but if this publication is the first of mine that you have read, this is the concept.

Every week from Monday all the way through to Saturday morning, I eat very clean. A typical day goes like this:

- Green juice, first thing in the morning – apple, root ginger, celery, lemon, kale, broccoli, spinach. Yes, this is a "Jim special," and it is for function and not taste. However, you would be surprised at how refreshing and easy this is to drink. I also believe that I am getting more fresh fruits and veggies into my body in one go than many people do in a week, and it's all happening before 8:00 am every morning.

- Next up is post-workout meal: porridge oats, natural peanut butter, and whey protein powder mixed with hot water. This is also more tasty than you would think. I use chocolate flavoured whey so that this tastes like a desert.

- Lunch time is normally a salad with iceberg lettuce, spring onion, red pepper, sauerkraut, and either chicken breast or mackerel fillet topped off with a light dressing. You can get some really low calorie dressings like ranch, Caesar, or blue cheese. It's worth looking into, but make sure to use these sparingly, since the recommended measure on most products is 15mm. You could also make your own dressing with a bit of extra virgin olive oil and balsamic vinegar.

- Evening meal is normally baked salmon fillet with mange tout, green beans, or broccoli and brown rice.

A fairly clean and healthy diet, right? So, it may surprise some to know that on some Saturdays, I have been known to eat two large stuffed crust pizzas and a bunch of chocolates whilst watching movies and not feel the least bit guilty about it. Why? Because I earned it, and as I had been so good with diet all week, that pizza tasted so much better than it would have if it was a part of my regular diet.

By adding a "Cheat night" in which you can choose to indulge in your favourite foods without feeling guilty about it, not only does it make your whole health, fitness, or weight-loss venture a lot more sustainable, it also adds a reward aspect; it takes away the guilt of eating naughty foods, gives you something to look forward to, and also helps you enjoy treats a whole lot more.

I would wait until I got to this stage in the game before adding a cheat night, as I would have already established some of the fundamental habits. My body should be responding to the new exercise, my metabolism would be in a better state to deal with a bit of junk food, and the likelihood that my mental state would crumble and push me back into eating junk food and turn me into Ben Stiller at the end of the movie *Dodgeball* would be far less.

I will close change #16 by saying that there are a few different ways to reward yourself in this manner, but this method has suited me the best. I would also mention that the longer you do this for, the less cravings for junk foods you will have, and if you do find yourself in a situation where you are unable to eat healthy food for a day or two, you will start to crave healthy salads, fresh fruits, and clean nutritious meals. I can attest to this.

Fitness Tip #17 (Exercise) – Join a gym!

Why?

Joining a gym is a very big step for a lot of people. I can recall when I first started training myself, I stepped into the weight room for the first time and had the feeling that everyone was looking down on me – the feeling of "not belonging" and the all-round discomforting sense of being a fish out of water. Even though I felt like this, I will admit that it was easier for me because I had joined with a friend, and I wasn't alone.

My personality is naturally introverted, and I have never liked being the centre of attention; this is why I have never taken for granted the effort that it takes for someone who is new to fitness to go to a gym, sign up, and walk into the weight room for the first time. Everyone who manages to break this mental barrier, step right out of their comfort zone, and take this action has 100% of my respect.

If you are in this situation yourself, and you can relate to this, please remember that everyone who looks like an "elite trainer" training at the gym started in the beginning at some point too, just as you did. They have their own goals and challenges, just as you do; they have a passion for their goals, just as you do; they are committed to their training, they take it seriously, and just like you, they have a personality outside of the gym.

In my experience, some of the most muscle bound, leanest, or strongest people in the gym are the most friendly and willing to help you out if they are asked. Sure, there are always a few exceptions to this rule as with all social, culture communities, but this should not be a reason to think twice about signing up at a gym.

Taking the above mentioned mental hurdles into consideration that many people have to overcome with this change, I would suggest that after signing up, you should start to work on establishing a gym routine.

Getting through the door to the gym is one thing, but knowing what to do when you are on the gym floor is another thing altogether. If you don't know what you are going to do each time you are there, it can make the mental challenge a whole lot tougher, even to the point that it may stop you from making the journey to the gym that day. This is a slippery slope.

For the first two weeks I suggest that –

- You visit the gym at least 3 times every week. Plan your training days with a view to use these three days as your "Gym days" for the foreseeable future.
- You choose one piece of cardio exercise equipment (Treadmill, cross trainer, rowing machine, stationary bike) and learn how to use it for steady state exercise. You can ask a member of the staff to demonstrate this on your first visit if you like.
- On each gym visit, go to your piece of equipment and spend thirty to forty-five minutes on it. "Steady state" is the key word here. It means that you maintain a constant pace that can be sustained for a long period. Think marathon, not sprint. The idea is to get used to the gym visits while not overexerting yourself. There will be plenty of opportunity to really test your abilities in the future.

This is a great way to get started and establish your gym visit routine; there are less variables that you have to worry about. Just concentrate on hitting your scheduled workout sessions, and the thirty to forty-five minutes cardio training will be a nice bonus. I would recommend doing this for a minimum of two weeks but not more than four weeks, since you will need to progress from this rather than risk this becoming your comfort zone.

Fitness Tip #18 (Exercise) – The next thing I would do is sign up for a challenge – a fun run, charity run, a hill walk challenge, cycle race, or a triathlon.

Why?
When looking at the fact that I would not even be a year into my new healthy way of living, and I would have only been a member of a gym for two weeks, it may seem extremely far-fetched that I would even consider signing up for an event like this.
This is the mentality that holds many people back. As a personal trainer, I had to resort to tricking a new client into doing thirty-minutes steady state cardio on an exercise bike because she was so

adamant that she couldn't do it that she wasn't even willing to try. In this session, I first "forgot" to start the stopwatch. I would randomly pause the timer for several minutes at a time without her knowing, and I managed to keep her talking and side-tracked until the thirty-minutes was up. At this point, I even had to tell her that we needed to stop as she would have kept on pedalling. During all of this, I had placed my clipboard over the timer that was actually part of the exercise bike, and when I showed her the "thirty six" minutes display, she was genuinely shocked. After this, my client was more than willing to try new challenges as she had left that menta; barrier destroyed and far behind.

Coming back to the fictional Jim now, at this stage, I would choose to sign up for a triathlon. Again, this may sound very unrealistic or a bit far-fetched, but it isn't at all.

When you hear the word "triathlon," it probably conjures up images of super-fit athletes competing against each other in a gruelling test of physical and mental stamina that is suited only to super-fit or hardened athletes.

You could look at a triathlon in this way, or I could lend you my set of "Jim's barrier-breaking, it-ain't-so-bad glasses." You can look at it as I would.

So, put them on and look at it again:

"Triathlon"

- It doesn't have to be a race; you can take your time.
- There are only three events in a triathlon.
- The triathlon doesn't have to be over large distances. You could even do a test triathlon in your gym that only takes thirty minutes.
- If there are no events in your local area, you could create your own personal triathlon to challenge yourself.

I'm going to need my glasses back now, or I might struggle to finish this book! Jokes aside, as you can see, if you look at any challenge for what it really is and not rely on the ethos commonly associated with it, there is a likelihood that it won't appear as daunting at all.

Aside from the physical benefits that will come from training for an event, there will be so much more to it. By committing to an actual date and training for the event, you will be giving yourself accountability, focus, and a reason to make your training progress. This will also be an enormous boon to your mental health as the challenge of the training will be an on-going development for your mental robustness.

When you decide to start looking for a physical event, I would suggest that you look for one around six months into the future. This way, you will have plenty of time to prepare. Once you find something, it will not be uncommon to think

"Okay, I'll start training for this and sign up near that time"

Does that say, "Yes! I'm committed to this, and I *will* do it!"?

Why is this a common response? It is because it's easy to waiver the commitment and self-doubt in us all, especially if you are new to physical challenges. The best way to achieve a goal is to go at it with 100% commitment and throw your heart and soul into making it happen.

To that end, once you find your challenge or event, sign up for it then and there.

Fitness Tip #19 (Exercise) – I would develop a good routine at the gym and train 3 times per week.

Why?

Now that I have a physical challenge planned, which is a far cry from my comfort zone, I will need to start thinking about the physical attributes that will help me get through.

A triathlon normally consists of three events – running, swimming, and cycling, and in order to make it easier for my body to deal with these, I will need to work on a few things.

I will need

- A basic foundation of cardiovascular stamina
- Good muscular stamina and strength, and it will help if I worked on lowering my body fat. I don't want to be lugging all that extra spud around with me.
- A positive attitude and a high level of commitment to the training and the challenge.

Since I started my cardio sessions all those weeks ago, I will be able to start jogging, adding some sprints, intervals, and experiment with the distance to develop my cardiovascular stamina. Although, I would probably need to work on my muscular endurance too.

Since I now have a gym membership and have been a member for two weeks, I would start to look at resistance training in order to introduce the development of my muscular strength and endurance.

My weapon of choice at this point would be to utilise a method of training known as "circuit training".

Circuit training would be ideal at this point since it would target every muscle in my body; it would be a big step up in my workouts, and the simple fact that training in a circuit style is fairly intense, there would be the added bonus of effective fat burning that will help shed that extra weight even more.

If you do decide to go down the route of circuit training, I would suggest that you take a look at one of my other books since I have taken care of everything in here. It's a fairly in-depth guide, but it has a lot of great tips for beginners:

<u>"Home Workout Circuit Training"</u>

Fitness Tip #20 (Mind-set) – I would learn the names and functions of muscle groups, and which resistance exercises work each muscle group.

Why?

If you really want to earn outstanding results and get what you pay for from your gym membership, you should learn the muscle groups and their functions. Like I have always said, this is a lifelong commitment. If you can build your knowledge of the functions of your body, you will not only learn to walk into any gym in the world, look at the equipment, and be able to figure out which machine does what or pick up a set of dumb-bells and train any muscle group that you wanted to with these weights, you will also learn a lot more about your own body, such as your strengths and weaknesses.

Knowledge of kinesiology is something that is truly worth investing your time in. If I were to start again, I would focus on learning a single muscle group every week. I would learn how to build it and how to shape it and actually test this out in the gym with different types of exercise at varying intensity and workloads. For example, on one of the weeks, I might choose to look into how the latissimus dorsi functions. These are the big muscles found on your back. I would learn that these muscles are among the biggest in the body and are responsible for pulling the arms in and back. I would come to know that there are several different ways by which I can target these muscles with barbells, machines, and bodyweight exercises. There are two common movements through which you can target these muscles in the gym: the rowing movements and the pull down movements. Once I have researched this muscle group, I would add a rowing exercise and a pull-down movement to my circuit session that week. The next week, I would swap these two exercises for another two in order to hit another muscle group that I had learned about.

This would mean that my circuit training sessions would have two extra exercises added to it; but these exercises would change every week to put another muscle group in the spotlight.

This is an excellent way to learn about training as it incorporates theory with practical. As I mentioned before, this fitness tip will also bring to your attention any weaknesses or indeed strengths that you were previously unaware of. The more you learn and experiment with this, the more valuable it will become.

Fitness Tip #21 (Exercise) – Next, I would swap one of my morning cardio sessions for a steady state jogging session every week.

Why?

A long steady state jogging session would give add some great benefits to my fitness goals. Not only would a steady state jog inject a huge boost to my fat burning goals, but I would also be working on my stamina levels in preparation for the triathlon challenge that I had signed up for.

The exercise choice of jogging or running can strike fear into the hearts of many beginners, and the mere thought of the effort that comes with getting ready for a jog, starting out on a thirty to forty minute exercise session such as jogging or running is enough to put many people off.

Since my morning walks have been going on for so long, the transition between brisk walking and jogging will be an easy one. If you have been following this plan so far, you may already be jogging in the mornings, or you may have made the transition from walking to jogging many weeks ago. If this is the case, you are ahead of the game and are doing an excellent job! But for those of us who have not made the transition yet, the time is now.

Steady state running or jogging basically means that you maintain one pace throughout your training session as opposed to interval training or sprint training.

The beauty of steady state jogging is that you can start off as slow as you like. If you have never jogged before, it can take a few weeks to find your ideal pace, but once you find this, you can build on it.

The main idea behind steady state running is that you can hold a conversation comfortably without gasping for breath whilst you are exercising. You should also be able to complete your entire route without stopping. If this is not happening, you should reduce your running pace.

One thing that I will mention at this point is that it can take up to ten minutes of jogging at the beginning of each run before your breathing finds its rhythm; so please be remember this before reducing your pace or giving up before you have even started. A good tweak is to spend a minute or two immediately before each cardio session breathing deeply and slowly. This will open up your lungs and prepare them for the upcoming session, and this should hopefully eliminate the whole breathing struggle at the start of the session.

If I were to start jogging as a complete beginner, I should be aware of the following few points:

- My first jogging session would use the route that I am familiar with (my usual walking route) and would set out from the start at a jogging pace that is not far off my usual brisk walking pace
- I would make sure that I have a good rhythm with my breathing. Believe it or not, this is something that can take a bit of concentration and practice to get right.
- I would monitor how I am feeling throughout the session – Am I feeling too out of breath? Is my back or knees hurting? Did I have to stop at any point because I was fighting for air?

If I had answered "Yes" to any of these questions, I would look into the reasons and identify the problems, but I would not let them put me off and stop me from progressing. If there is a problem, I would consider fixing it.

If you follow this change and find that your back, knees, or any other part of your body gives you any kind of pain, it may be down to your running technique or posture. If you were too out of breath, it may be down to your breathing rhythm or your jogging speed may be too fast. These are just a few of the common snags that crop up with beginners to running and jogging. If you do run into these and would like a more comprehensive guide on how to overcome these glitches along with more practical advice, I have written another book titled *Marathon Training & Distance Running* that you might want to check out. This is a beginners guide, so it would be most useful to guys who are just starting out.

Fitness Tip #22 (Exercise) – For my next change, I would substitute one of my morning cardio sessions with a swimming session.

Why?

As mentioned earlier, this is still the first year of my new lifestyle, and I think that it would be a great idea to try a variety of different exercise options. Swimming could be my go-to cardio choice, but I wouldn't know until I have tried it.

Swimming also fits in nicely since it is one of the events in the triathlon; so, this gives me an extra measure of accountability.

I appreciate that swimming is not the most convenient of exercise choices for most people, since not everyone may not have a swimming pool at their doorstep. This will take up more time than a simple walking or jogging session since there would be the added journey to and from the pool; so for most, this may be too time restrictive to implement in the morning before work. However, if you would like to use this change in your own plan, you may wish to try swimming one evening after work or even add a session on the weekend.

This is how I would approach a swimming session:

- I would have a target distance that I intend to reach. The swimming pool that I would use is twenty five meters long; so, I would aim for 20 lengths to start with. (Please remember that as an individual, and due to years of positive thinking, I am sometimes over-ambitious. So, I may well fail at hitting this target, but I would always be back to try again until the target was reached). If you decide to go down the swimming path, I would encourage you to also be over-ambitious too. Who knows, you might even surprise yourself by comfortably reaching your target in your first attempt.

- I would decide on a stroke that I was going to cover the distance in. Hands down, this would be the breast stroke. Not only does breast stroke engage nearly all the muscles in the body, it is also a good choice for long sustained or steady state pacing, which means that it should take a lot longer for your body to become fatigued than a stroke like the front crawl or the butterfly would.

- I would find out the opening time of my swimming pool of choice and make sure that my sessions would be at a time when the pool is least busy; or if there are any timings when the pool is reserved for lane swimming only. This way, I would be among like-minded people and would have less distraction and more focus.

I understand that this is a big ask for many people, since it is probably the most restrictive fitness tip that I have mentioned so far. If you are following this plan to the letter, but there is no way that you can implement this, you may want to try another cardio based exercise such as bike riding or boxing. There is a whole lot that you can do with a punch bag and a stopwatch. Please feel free to drop me an email if you are struggling for ideas, and I'll do my best to help you come up with some ideas that suit you better.

Fitness Tip #23 (Exercise) – I would substitute one of my morning cardio sessions with a sprint training session once per week.

Why?
All of the cardio based exercise suggested so far was focused on fat burning and steady state. This means that the body will adapt to this type of training and develop for this type of activity. Of course, this is great, and it is exactly what we are looking to do, but there are other training methods out there that would give us a better balance.
If you look at the most extreme examples of different running conditioning by looking at the physiques of the best sprinters and the best long distance runners, and you compare the two, you will notice it very clearly. Usain Bolt is a fairly muscled guy; he is built for speed and explosive power, and he has trained with this in mind. When sprinting, his body only has to work for around ten seconds in an event. However, if you look at Mo Farah, you will see that he is extremely lean and doesn't carry a lot of muscle mass; he is built for stamina and trains to work for events that last for much longer periods.

Sprinting and long-distance running are very different beasts. Some people are naturally built for one rather than the other. Jogging or long distance running is a progression from walking, and as a result, it will feel more comfortable to go for a jog rather than a sprint. However, sprint training can really help with lung capacity and help develop power while challenging the muscles in a whole new way.

This is where I would start with sprint training:

- Once every week, I would find a fifty to one hundred meter stretch of flat uninterrupted land. There are plenty of quiet fields and parks where I am, but if you live in a built-up area, you could use a quiet road or footpath, empty car park, disused railway line – there is always a way!
- I would warm up with a light ten to fifteen minute jog and stretch out my hamstrings, quads, and calves, making sure that I am suitably warm (If it is possible for you to do this sprint training mid-way through your usual cardio route, it would be ideal). I would then sprint the length of my planned out track and slowly jog back.
- Once I have reached the starting point again, I would immediately sprint the route again and repeat until I have completed five sprints in total.
- Five sprints would be my starting point, and I would add another sprint every two weeks if I wished to develop my sprinting ability further.

A word of warning – if you are not used to sprint training, you can very quickly become exhausted, feel sick, struggle to breath, and your upper leg muscles may feel like they've turned to jelly, but the more you train like this, the better your body will cope with it. This means that the training is beginning to have its effect, and you are getting better. So, if you do decide to take up this challenge, and you feel like your world has ended after a few sprints, please don't be put off; it is totally normal, and you will get better the more you train in this way.

Fitness Tip #24 (Mind-set) – The next thing that I would do is to take stock of my progress. What have I achieved, what did I enjoy, and what do I want to pursue?

Why?

At this point, it would almost be a year since I started, and I would have been through a lot, physically and mentally. I would have learned much about myself; my strengths, weaknesses, what I enjoyed, and what I didn't want to do again. I may have found a fitness niche that I really wanted to become good at or even found that I was a natural at something.

Whatever happened throughout this year, I would have laid, or began to lay, the foundations of my future fitness and lifestyle path. I would have the experience of the training, and the feeling of accomplishment, the development of mental strength, not to mention the physical changes that would be evident for all to see.

When you follow your plan, there are more than likely going to be some changes along the way; little wobbles or outright road blocks. Unforeseen circumstances are a part of life, and so too a part of fitness goals and development. It's very rare that the road will be a straight one with zero obstructions, but if you want to arrive at your destination, you need to keep going, or you will never get there. At this point, I would look back and note any problems that I had since the beginning. I would write down all the times that things didn't go to plan – Did I cheat on my diet? Did I not learn enough new healthy cooking recipes that caused me to want to eat the bad stuff? Did I not progress as much as I should have on my resistance training or cardio? Did I skip lots of training sessions?

Anything that was not a part of the original plan, that caused detriment to the overall goal, would be noted here.

I would also make a note of anything that wasn't on the original plan but had caused positive development. Maybe I had decided to start jogging earlier on in my plan and had to miss out this change when it was due as it was already in progress. Maybe I switched a change one week because my goals had changed, and I wanted to make my future progression align with my new goals a bit better? These are all positive things that may have caused me to deviate, and these changes are the ones that help to really pave the way for future goals. Thus, they should be recognised.

I would suggest that you take some time to think about what has happened, and how it has affected you. Take some time between this change and the next one to really identify what worked with you and what didn't; what you would like to continue doing, and what you really don't want to. These are some more things to think about to help you get started:

- Are you more likely to enjoy a cardio-based fitness routine, or do you prefer lifting heavy weights?
- Were you able to fit in any exercise sessions into your daily routine easily, or was it a bit of a struggle?
- Are there any foods that you didn't really like or did you find some really healthy, guilt-free cooking recipes that will help you with your fitness goals?
- Is there anything that you would like to try that you haven't already?

I would suggest that you take the next two weeks to really think about this, as the deeper you go, the better prepared you will be for the next fitness tip.

Fitness Tip #25 (Mind-set) - For the final change at the end of my first year, I would plan for the next year.

Why?

There are a few reasons why I would plan out my next twenty-five changes. Many people would think that the number one reason is to "keep me working on my new healthy lifestyle" or "to keep me interested so that I don't slip back into my old ways." This is a very good reason, but it slips into the number two position, right behind "stopping progression".

If you have followed a weight-loss, muscle-toning, or general healthy living plan for almost a year, although it is still possible to slip right back and go downhill, it is unlikely. You will have established plenty of good habits. However, there is always the whole "homeostasis" function that is ready to jump in and stop any progression.

After a year, if you are happy with the new you, great! You can go ahead and train and live to maintain. However, I would always suggest that you do challenge yourself at least once every month with something that is not a part of your usual routine. For example, if you have taken to strength training in the gym as your preferred resistance training choice, you may want to throw in a good circuit training session once a while that challenges you in different ways, or you may want to go for a sprint session. Likewise, if you are into steady state running, you may want to throw in a gym session that focuses on strength training once in a while. Doing this will keep your body from developing a state of homeostasis in which your fitness level and motivation may stagnate.

The last change of your first twenty-five fitness tips should be used to plan out another new beginning. This may be easier, and it may have changes and tweaks on a less frequent timescale; but, it will probably be more focused on certain areas. At this point in fictional Jim's progression, I know that he would like to focus on building muscle and would like to plan his next year dedicated to bodybuilding. That motivational picture of Arnold we spoke of earlier would almost definitely get him motivated enough to want to earn what he had earned in the picture. The physical and mental challenges that fictional Jim had overcame so far in his fitness and lifestyle journey would give him the belief that it is indeed possible for him to achieve great bodybuilding results. Luckily for fictional Jim, there is a great plan that's been mapped out for exactly this, and its already waiting for him. It's called *Jim's weight training and bodybuilding guide"*, written by some guy called "Jim"! What are the odds?

Of course, everyone is different, and the idea of bodybuilding will be far from many peoples aspirations. Nevertheless, if you can plan your next stage to incorporate exercise that you enjoy, food that you like to eat, and goals that motivate you, you will have done an excellent job in your first year, and you can look forward to more rewards going forward.

This can take a bit of time and effort, and it may feel like a big pointless chore, but planning really is invaluable. Once it's done, it's done, and you will have a guide to keep you on track when times get tough, and you are less likely to lose your way.

So plan and plan good.

NINE

BE AMAZED AT YOUR ACHIEVEMENTS

When you reach this point, whether you have followed the fitness tips exactly, tweaked them slightly, or made your own list entirely, you will have been through many challenges, and you will have learned a lot about yourself. You will be physically and mentally stronger and may even have inspired others to follow in your footsteps. You will have achieved a great deal.

You will have experience of several types of exercise, and this will have given you a good reference as to where you want to focus your efforts for the next year. After this, you may enjoy cross-country running more and may wish to peruse that. You may also find that you are naturally strong when it comes to resistance training and wish to spend more time in the free weights area; or you may even find that you have a natural ability for long distance swimming or running. As you can see, by spending your first year building your fitness, exercise, and lifestyle routines by adding all of these different activities, you are likely to lean towards certain exercise methods more than others. This way, moving onto your second year, you will be more equipped, focused, and are likely to even have fresh ambitious goals.

This is the start of great things, and if you have managed to get through the first year, I can almost guarantee that you will never look back again. This will change your whole life; so, make this next year the one where you develop your mind and body into something that you are proud of and will drive you forward to become more than you ever thought was possible.

ARE YOU READY TO COMMIT?

FINAL THOUGHTS

Can you do it? Can you plan a whole year of positive changes and see them through? Of course, you can. The real question is – do you want it bad enough to make a few sacrifices and go through a few uncomfortable times?

If you are the type of person who's no stranger to takeaway food, high-calorie/low-nutrition snacks, lead an inactive lifestyle, and are becoming increasingly overweight and unfit, then it will be more difficult. However, you will benefit the most.

One of the most resounding long-term and life-changing alterations in you will be the shift from your body craving fatty non-nutritious food and shuddering at the thought of exercise to the need for healthy, fresh food and regular physical activity.

I know this because I have lived it first-hand. There was a time in my life when I followed a fairly unhealthy standard of living. I was a lot younger, had been convinced by some bad advice and thought that it was the way to go. I will briefly summarise my weekly food and exercise habits to outline my experience.

The bottom line was that I believed putting on serious mass to become a great bodybuilder was to eat absolutely everything, double up on my food intake, and rest my body as much as possible to the point that if I didn't need to stand up, I would lie down to conserve as many calories as possible. Yes, this is absolutely ridiculous, and as a fitness author, I am slightly embarrassed by it. Nevertheless, it was just one of the valuable lessons I had learnt on my personal journey.

I fell into the habit of eating large portions of high-calorie food and didn't really look at nutrition closely. On top of this, I would drink high-calorie weight gainer drinks a few times per day. I would make a big lasagne once every week and eat a huge portion of this with a big chunk of crusty white bread and butter. It was also a regular thing to have a night when I would eat two large chicken kebabs and fries, a Chinese takeaway night when I would order two different main courses, and on Sunday night, it was "Maccy dees". This would be eating two large burger meals. I would also have nights when I didn't go to the gym, and I would immerse myself in my favourite online game and eat a big bag of peanut MnMs and drink cappuccinos. This was just my evening eating habits; so, you can imagine how bad the rest of the time was. I would, however, drive to the gym five times per week and train with heavy weights, but this didn't really help with my general health. There are far better and more efficient ways to approach the goals that I wanted. I finally started to change my ways when my bodyweight reached sixteen stone. I have always been a skinny guy, and this is attributed to my genetics. I was never meant to weigh that much, and I really started to struggle with normal tasks like putting on my socks or walking up the stairs. My training partner even started to get worried in our training sessions when I would finish a heavy set of leg presses and fight for air. I must have been quite the picture of health.

Despite my training sessions, I was fat and unfit.

Its many years later now, and I am healthy and lean. Going back to the original point of this anecdote, I can say that if I had decided to make all of the necessary diet, training, and lifestyle changes that I follow today in one go when I was at my most unhealthy and unfit state. My body would have an enormous shock, and I would struggle. It would not be long before cravings for chocolate and large portions of unhealthy food hit me, and these cravings would hit hard. I would struggle with the training that I do now if I could do a full session at all, and this would all be because I had trained my body to live and function in a certain way. These days, if I go a day or two without fresh fruits and vegetables, don't drink enough water, overeat, eat too much food that's low in good nutrition, or I miss a training session, my body starts to struggle. I will crave for a green juice or a fresh tuna or salmon salad; I will need to go to the gym and push my body physically. This is because I have trained my body to accept this as the normal functionary levels. This is known as homeostasis.

Whatever lifestyle you live, your body will adapt to it. Everyone has a routine or lifestyle that they choose to follow; whether this is a clean, healthy, balanced routine or a pizza-fuelled, online gaming joyride.

Changing your body's homeostasis is tough, and that statement stands on a two-way street basis; so, if you can change from unhealthy to healthy, it will be hard to go back, and this is the message at the heart of this guide. Everyone wants to live a healthier lifestyle, and hopefully, this guide will help you to make the shift with minimal disruption.

I love to hear of people's success, and it has been so great to hear from readers and listeners of my books. To know that my work is having a positive impact on people's lives keeps me going, and it saddens me to think that I was nearly talked out of committing to the goal of writing fitness advice for a living. In fact, if I had listened to everyone that said I couldn't or shouldn't do something that I planned to do, or if I had been put off by someone who laughed at me and my plans, I would not have joined the army, I would not have attempted airborne training, I would not have quit a job that I hated to earn a living from the internet, and I would not have competed in a bodybuilding competition, to name a few things. Therefore, if you have an ambitious fitness goal, or any other goal for that matter, I would suggest that you commit to it and go at it with full conviction, not letting anyone stand in your way. People may laugh at your plans to run a marathon or compete in a triathlon; they may try to convince you to downscale your ambition, but if you let someone else influence your true goals, you may be missing out on seeing your true potential.

I, for one, feel that its okay to fail; I can live with that. But, I would not be able to live with myself if I never tried.

"If you shoot for the moon and miss, you will end up among the stars"

Are you ready to commit to a tough year? It will be hard, but it will give you so much more than just positive physical change. You will learn about yourself; you will have a sense of achievement that cannot be explained to anyone until they have earned it and felt it for themselves; you will be mentally robust, and you will have self-respect and respect from your peers. However, one of the greatest achievements in my opinion is that you will inspire others to follow in your footsteps and actually be instrumental in changing their lives. In doing so, this will have a knock-on effect, such as a domino rally or ripples on a pond from a stone splash.

I truly hope that you find this guide useful, and as always, I am more than happy to help out further where I can. If you need someone to bounce some ideas off, or if you have any struggles, physically or mentally, I would be happy to give you my thoughts. So, give me a shout out.

Thanks so much for reading, and I wish you the very best with your future plans.

All the best,

Jim

(James Atkinson)

FITNESS & EXERCISE
MOTIVATION

I would like to leave you with an excerpt from one of my other books that complements the book you've just finished reading. It will help you further develop your training. *"Fitness & Exercise Motivation"* was written for the beginner to fitness or anyone who has ever struggled to achieve real fitness results. These two books go hand in hand, so either can be the sequel or prequel to the other.

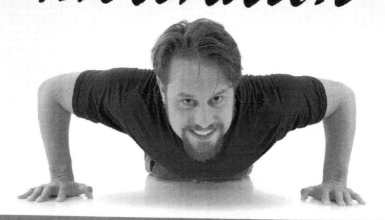

JAMES ATKINSON

FITNESS & EXERCISE
Motivation

FITNESS SUCCESS TIPS FOR MIND-SET DEVELOPMENT
AND PERSONAL FITNESS PLANNER CREATION

IT STARTS WITH A REASON

Whenever anyone decides to take on a fitness venture, new diet, or healthy lifestyle change, there is always a trigger. If there wasn't a reason to do this, why would it even cross your mind?

Most people who decide that they want to start a physical training routine or health diet will want to do this because of the way they feel. It might be that they feel overweight and unattractive, and when they see themselves in the mirror, they don't like what they see. On the other hand, it might be that they are training for a sporting event and bodily changes need to be made.

The point is; if you are looking to start a new fitness regime, there is always a reason.

Most people, including my past self, overlook this extremely powerful tool called 'Reason' by having a *subliminal* reason; that is, they don't exactly know what their reason is. This can really weaken their chances of success at the subconscious state.

When I look back on my own personal experiences today, I can identify my reasons for doing the things I did. I can explain my reasoning for the big choices I made. But at some points in my life, I could not.

I was in my late twenties when I first started to utilize this tool, and it was actually someone else who set me on this way of thinking. I had gone into bodybuilding in a big way since I left the army several years earlier, and I had wanted to compete in a bodybuilding show for the last few years.

One day, I was speaking to a work colleague during break whilst showing him some pictures of some of the guys who trained at my gym and who had already competed in bodybuilding shows. My work colleague didn't have the slightest interest in fitness or physical training, and I should've probably been chatting to him about something else. But when someone has a passion for a goal or a hobby, they tend to share it with everyone they meet, and I had gone very much down this rabbit hole.

As he flicked through the picture gallery on my phone, you could follow his thought process by looking at his face. The subjects of these photographs were of men who were wearing nothing but a set of extra small posing trunks. They were smeared in deep, dark, fake tans with hard, lean, muscular physiques; and to top it off, they were all striking some kind of "show off" pose.

As he handed my phone back to me, with a grimace on his face, he said:

"Why do you want to look like that?"

In my infinite wisdom, I replied in my typical light-hearted style, "Chicks dig muscles, don't they?"

Although my answer didn't do a lot for the reputation of the bodybuilding community, it was, no doubt, the kind of answer that my colleague had come to expect of me, as I am a bit of a joker anyway. It was obvious that he wasn't very impressed with my plans and I realized that the discussion had come to an end, so we steered the conversation in another direction.

On my way home from work that night, when I had plenty of *thinking time* in my car, I thought about his question again.

Why do you want to look like that?

Now that I was alone with my thoughts, I could be perfectly honest with myself without being scrutinized by anyone but yours truly. So, what were the real reasons?

As I made the forty-five-minute car journey back home, I set about questioning myself and searching to find the real reasons that I wanted to contest in a bodybuilding show. Most people don't want to do this kind of thing so there must be something that had caused me to want to take up the challenge.

After being brutally honest with myself and facing the potentially humiliating truth, I came up with the real reasons. I was able to identify that wanting to compete in a bodybuilding show was a progression from overcoming an inferiority complex that I had when I was in my younger, more influential years, and an unfulfilled need to overcome a physical and mental challenge.

But if I had said that to my work colleague earlier, he would have probably been left speechless as it would have been way out of character for me to confess such a thing. And, in all fairness, earlier that day, I didn't realize that was the answer, either.

When I was younger, I was always a small kid. I really wanted to be the Johna Lomu or Scott Gibbs on the rugby pitch and destroy

85

my opponents with my awesome power, speed and bulk. When I watched these guys play rugby on television for their respective countries, I developed goose bumps as I watched them knock other players down, break out of multiple tackle attempts and carry the ball across the try line to lead their team to victory. But I would only ever be able to imagine what it felt like to be them. I was too small and weak to be anything but a liability on the rugby pitch, so I had to settle for being a substitute player. Until I found that I could work on my strength and size using a weight-lifting routine!

Many years later, after overcoming many more challenges and learning some valuable lessons along the way that, in turn, shaped my personality and changed me into a different person altogether, I would jump at any opportunity to prove that I could overcome tough physical and mental challenges.

I hit bodybuilding hard, and, after a few years, I actually looked like a bodybuilder. But to really reach my potential, I would have to strip away as much fat as possible, and the only real way to do this is with some solid accountability. What better way to put yourself under pressure to achieve a goal than to have a timescale and strong reason to accomplish that goal. If I were to commit to a bodybuilding competition and the day of the competition finally came, I would be standing on a stage in nothing but a tight thong, and in front of several hundred people. Now, if you were going to be doing that, you would really want to look your best!

On that drive home, I found out a lot about myself and it was as a result of being true to a simple question that my work colleague had thrown at me.

At that point, I committed to the bodybuilding competition. Although it was only months away, and I could bow out at any time, I decided I wasn't going to. I would see it through to the end and stand on that stage looking the best that I possibly could.

This appears to be the underlying reason that would carry me to the finish line. But there were other powerful reasons working their magic in the background, too:

- I was working a job that was not suited to me and really needed a challenge outside of work.
- I wanted to push myself to see how far I could go.
- I didn't want to be the average Joe who lifted weights and had some size.
- I didn't want to be the guy who says, "I thought about doing a bodybuilding show once." I wanted to be the guy who says, "I did a bodybuilding show once, and here's my trophy."
- I wanted to add *bodybuilding competition* to my "Achieved" list.
- I had been out of the army for several years and needed the challenge of hardship that comes with competition prep, so that I could taste the sweetest of sweetness after the long months of sour when the competition was over. (This is an awesome feeling!)
- I wanted an epic Facebook profile picture ☺

So, as you can see, finding a powerful reason or a number of reasons to take you beyond your own targets to achieve personal victories is not just a surface thought process. To get the best out of this tool, you must delve deep into your soul and really try to hit the nail on the head. And the more honest that you can be with yourself, the more of an accurate truth you will find.

Remember that you are the only person who knows your real reasons for wanting to change your fitness levels; so it pays to be as critical as you can be with yourself. This is how the most powerful reasons come to light.

If the reason isn't strong enough to drive you forward and force you to your feet when the challenges of your goal bring you to your knees, then the reason isn't good enough! Everyone's reasons will be different, and what one person might find ridiculous or even comical, might be strong enough to drive another person past limits beyond their own comprehension.

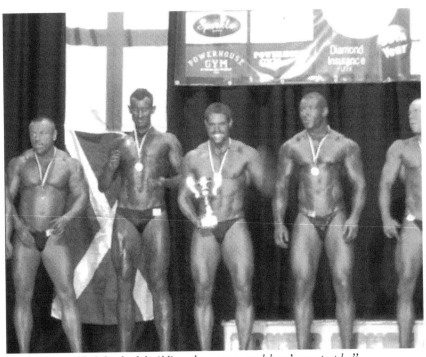

"I did a bodybuilding show once, and here's my trophy"

WHAT DID YOU THINK?

I am always eager to hear what you think of my books and exercise routines.

I would really appreciate it if you left a review and rating on the online retail store from which you made this purchase and tell others about your experience.

Please take a few moments to do this if you have enjoyed this book.

Just a few sentences and a few minutes of your time would help me out enormously, and I would be more grateful than you will know.

Thanks for the feedback! ☺

ALSO BY JAMES ATKINSON

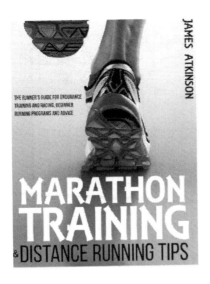

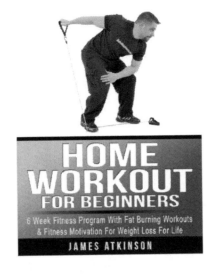

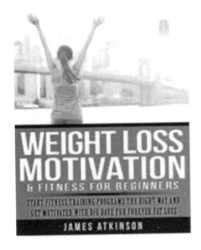

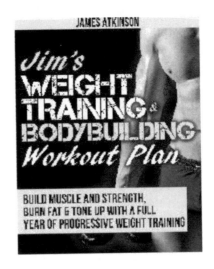

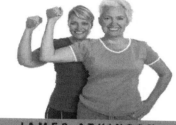

FITNESS FOR
WOMEN
OF ANY AGE

WOMEN'S HEALTH AND FITNESS ROUTINES,
CELLULITE AND WEIGHT LOSS TO TONING AND SCULPTING

JAMES ATKINSON

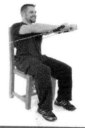

TOTAL FITNESS
— FOR —
WHEELCHAIR USERS

WHEELCHAIR WORKOUT, FITNESS TIPS FOR
FAT LOSS AND MUSCLE TONE

JAMES ATKINSON

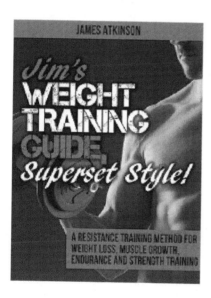

JAMES ATKINSON

Jim's
WEIGHT TRAINING GUIDE
Superset Style!

A RESISTANCE TRAINING METHOD FOR
WEIGHT LOSS, MUSCLE GROWTH,
ENDURANCE AND STRENGTH TRAINING

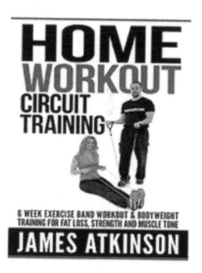

HOME
WORKOUT
CIRCUIT
TRAINING

6 WEEK EXERCISE BAND WORKOUT & BODYWEIGHT
TRAINING FOR FAT LOSS, STRENGTH AND MUSCLE TONE

JAMES ATKINSON

CONNECT WITH JIM

Visit Jim's blog for more great advice on diet, training, healthy recipes, motivation, and more: www.jimshealthandmuscle.com

Get regular updates on Facebook when you "like" and "follow" Jim's pages here:

Facebook.com/JimsHealthandMuscle
Facebook.com/SwapFat4Fit

Catch the trends. Follow Jim on Twitter here:

@JimsHM

Make some notes here. What's your plan?

Make some notes here. What's your plan?

Make some notes here. What's your plan?